TENDON TRANSFERS TO RESTORE
OPPOSITION OF THE THUMB

TENDON TRANSFERS TO RESTORE OPPOSITION OF THE THUMB

J. M. RAMSELAAR M. D.

H. E. STENFERT KROESE N.V. | LEIDEN 1970

ISBN-13: 978-90-207-0220-0   e-ISBN-13: 978-94-011-6780-2
DOI: 10.1007/978-94-011-6780-2

Library of Congress Catalog Card Number 79-125542

CONTENTS

INTRODUCTION

In man and some of the apes, the thumb has the function of a contra-finger. This function is made possible by a great freedom of movement of the first metacarpal and a highly developed and differentiated thumb musculature. The grasp function of the hand is dependent on the oppositional capacity and adductive power of the thumb, and is severely limited by a paralysis or dysfunction of the intrinsic thumb muscles. Whereas loss of the function of the adductor pollicis can be partially compensated for by the adductive action of the extensor pollicis longus, in paralysis or dysfunction of the radial thenar muscles compensation can only be provided by surgery.

Since 1918, many methods of tendon transfer have been described for the restoration of thumb opposition, all of which bring about an improvement of the grasp function, albeit to different degrees. These methods vary in the selection of the motor, the direction of pull of the tendon, the use of a fulcrum, and the mode of insertion. The highly effective method of Bunnell (1938) is often used as the standard procedure. With this method, the flexor superficialis tendon of the ring finger is looped around the tendon of the flexor carpi ulnaris and passed subcutaneously across the thenar eminence, after which it is fixed on the thumb at the level of the metacarpo-phalangeal joint.

In the reconstruction of the thumb opposition, however, a standard procedure often cannot be applied, because the muscle-tendon unit usually used for this purpose has been damaged or because the transfer route is blocked by scar tissue. When the loss of opposition is incomplete, a simpler tendon transfer will usually suffice. In practice, each opposition reconstruction requires that a choice be made from a series of transfer possibilities. Problems arise in cases with a lesion of the median and ulnar nerves, in which the injury usually renders several muscles and tendons unsuitable for a tendon transfer, while a suitable muscle-tendon unit must be found for correction of the loss of the opposition, the disturbed flexion pattern of the fingers, and sometimes also for the abduction of the index finger and the adduction of the thumb. In such cases an alternative solution is the static fixation of the thumb in the position of opposition.

In this thesis the possibilities for a dynamic restoration of thumb opposition are discussed, and illustrated on the basis of eight selected cases, each of which is representative of a number of aspects that can influence the choice of the method used to effect the restoration.

The reconstructive treatment of loss of opposition demands in the very first place an understanding of the functional anatomy of the thumb and the functional defect occurring when the innervation of the intrinsic thumb muscles is disturbed. Both these subjects are therefore discussed in the opening chapters.

CHAPTER I

FUNCTIONAL ANATOMY OF THE THUMB

The most characteristic and elementary movement of the thumb is opposition. In this movement the thumb is placed such that its distal volar side is diametrically opposite the distal volar side of one of the other fingers. The movement by which the thumb returns to the position it assumes in the open hand is called retroposition. The term opposition therefore concerns a complex of fundamental movements in the three thumb joints: the interphalangeal, the metacarpo-pha-langeal, and the carpo-metacarpal. The share taken by the trapezio-scaphoideal joint in the opposition movement is relatively unimportant (Bunnell, 1956).

Movements in the carpo-metacarpal joint

The movements of the first metacarpal are described in this study in relation to the corresponding movements of the other fingers. Many authors, however, take the anatomic position as the point of reference for defining all fundamental movements and therefore interchange the names of the movements of the first metacarpal, here termed flexion-extension and abduction-adduction. To avoid confusion at least partially, some French authors call flexion and extension of the first metacarpal '*antepulsion*' and '*rétropulsion*' (Adam, 1941; Rabischong, 1964; Valentin, 1966).

The distal joint surface of the trapezium has in principle two curvatures, one convex and the other concave. The axis of the concave curvature runs roughly parallel to the surface of the palm of the hand, the axis of the convex curvature almost at right angles to it. Abduction and adduction of the first metacarpal therefore take place in a direction roughly perpendicular to the surface of the palm, flexion and extension in a direction approximately parallel to it.

During circumduction óf the thumb the metacarpal head moves along an almost circular ellipse. The axis of the cone having this ellipse as base and the carpo-metacarpal joint as vertex can be taken as the starting-point for the description of the movements of the first metacarpal (Fig. 1).

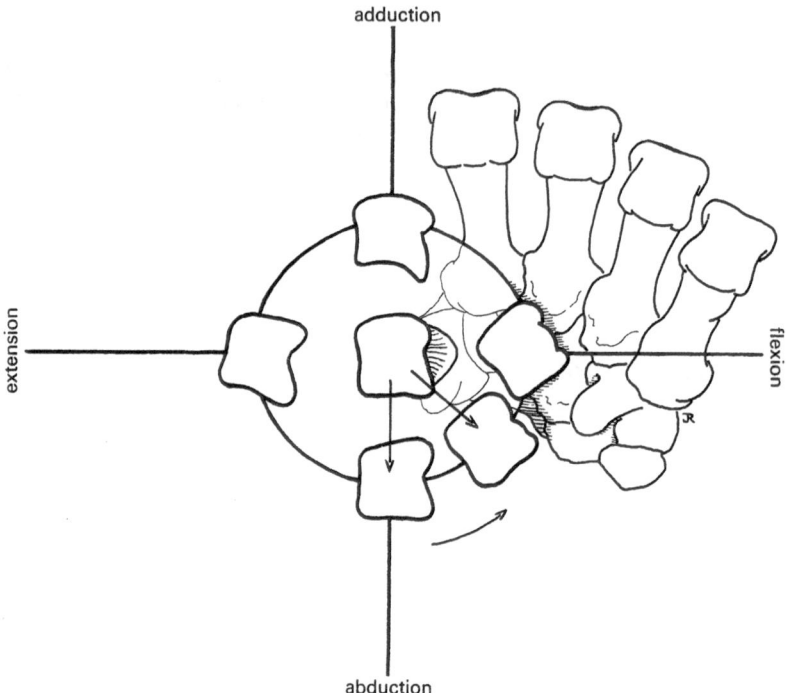

Fig. 1. Movements of the first metacarpal; opposition via direct and indirect pathways.

When the first metacarpal is in the central or neutral position, the carpo-metacarpal joint has a relatively great passive mobility due to the incongruence of the articular surfaces and the laxity of the ligaments (Fick, 1911). Haines (1944) distinguished in these ligaments a dorsal oblique, a volar oblique, and a radial carpo-metacarpal ligament in addition to a dorsal and a volar intermetacarpal ligament (Fig. 2).

When the first metacarpal is in abduction or adduction, part of this ligament complex is tightened and the joint surfaces are congruent. The stability thus achieved in both positions is very important for the grasp function of the hand.

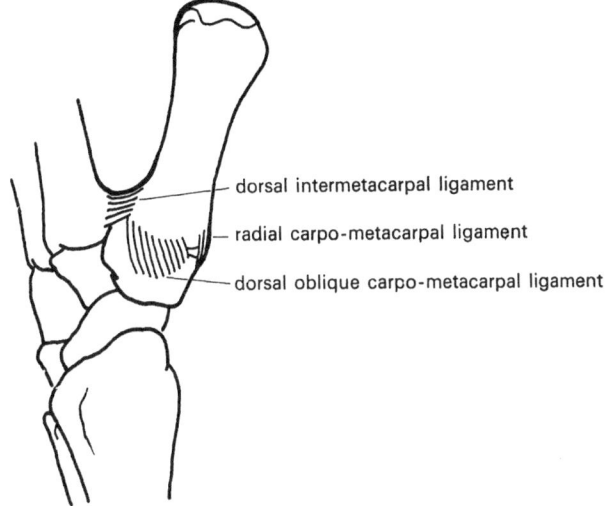

dorsal intermetacarpal ligament

radial carpo-metacarpal ligament

dorsal oblique carpo-metacarpal ligament

Fig. 2. Carpo-metacarpal joint of the left thumb; dorso-radial view.

In flexion and extension of the first metacarpal, the ligaments are initially relaxed. Toward the end of the flexion movement, according to Haines, the dorsal oblique carpo-metacarpal and the dorsal intermetacarpal ligaments tighten, as a result of which the first metacarpal is drawn into a pronation of about 30°, and toward the end of the extension movement the volar oblique carpo-metacarpal ligament becomes taut, resulting in a supination of about 15°. The arrangement of the ligaments around the first carpo-metacarpal joint and their guiding actions at the extremes of flexion and extension, as described by Haines, could not be entirely confirmed in a ligamentous preparation (Landsmeer, 1969) and requires further study. The total flexion-extension range of the metacarpal bone averages about 55°, the abduction-adduction movement 45°. The individual variations are considerable, however.

At opposition of the thumb, the first metacarpal comes into abduction, flexion, and pronation. Napier (1955) suggests that the opposition position of the first metacarpal can in principle be reached along two pathways: the *direct* and the *indirect* (Fig. 1).

If the indirect route is followed, the first metacarpal makes an abduction movement in the carpo-metacarpal joint, followed by a circumduction in the ulnar direction. This detour is unavoidably accompanied by a medial rotation (pronation), since according to a mechanical principle of synovial joints circumduction always involves some rotation, the so-called 'conjunct rotation'. This conjunct rotation is most effective in a saddle joint (MacConaill, 1946). According to Napier, during circumduction the dorsal oblique carpo-metacarpal ligament remains tense.

The alternative route is the direct one in which the first metacarpal is brought into opposition from the neutral position via the shortest path. In this case a rotator must bring about the pronation ('adjunct rotation') in the carpo-metacarpal joint. It may be assumed that this rotator role is filled by the opponens pollicis. During this opposition movement the dorsal oblique carpo-metacarpal ligament remains lax as long as pronation has not been completed.

According to Napier, the size of the object to be grasped determines which route is followed in the grasping movement. We assign more importance to his supposition that an opposition position can be achieved with a stable as well as with a rather unstable carpo-metacarpal joint.

Landsmeer (1962) classified the prehensile movements of the hand according to two basic patterns; the *power grip* and *precision handling*. In the former the object is grasped and held between the fingers (and thumb) and the middle hand, i.e. the thenar, hypothenar, and palmar delta. When the object is spherical, the thumb is in opposition. If it is cylindrical, then depending on the size of the circumference the thumb is held in either opposition or adduction. During precision handling the object is taken between the tips of the fingers and moved or manipulated between the fingers, for which opposition of the thumb is imperative. Power is hardly exerted in precision handling. The thumb remains in movement, varying from index finger to little finger opposition and from the 'flexed' to the 'extended' position of opposition. Great stability of the carpo-metacarpal joint will not be required or even desirable for this work. It therefore seems conceivable that for the power grip the indirect opposition route is followed and for precision handling the direct route.

On the whole, these two routes should be seen as the extremes of a range of opposition routes with combinations of conjunct and adjunct rotation, in the sense that precision handling can also be performed with power and the power grip with precision. The distinction between a direct and an indirect route acquires clinical significance when the abductor pollicis brevis and the opponens pollicis no longer function, while the abductor pollicis longus and flexor pollicis brevis are intact.

Movements in the metacarpo-phalangeal joint

In opposition of the thumb the proximal phalanx is brought into abduction, pronation, and flexion. The extent of these movements is dependent on the shape and size of the object to be grasped and on the position it must assume in the hand. These movements are most pronounced when the tip of the thumb approaches the base of the little finger. For opposition with respect to the index finger, only a minor amount of abduction and flexion in the metacarpo-phalangeal joint is required. If the object has a large circumference, this joint is even extended.

When the thumb is in adduction, the metacarpo-phalangeal joint is slightly flexed or extended and slightly adducted.

The total abduction-adduction movement of the proximal phalanx averages 25°, the rotation 30° (Fick, 1911).

The range of flexion-extension shows wide individual variation. Harris and Joseph (1949) found that flexion varied from 5° to 88° and extension from 34° to 48° hyperextension. The other movements in the metacarpo-phalangeal joint differ less strongly among individuals. The cause of these differences lies in the shape of the joint surfaces – round or flat – or in the tension of the joint capsule, or both (Joseph, 1951). The flat type of joint occurs in only 10 per cent of the cases. This has some clinical importance: in a round joint type with a lax capsule, the stability of the metacarpo-phalangeal joint depends entirely on muscle action.

Limitation of the flexion-extension movement in the metacarpo-phalangeal joint seldom means a substantial loss of thumb function.

The presence of sesamoid bones in the capsule of the metacarpo-phalangeal joint has little functional importance. In the evolutionary sense, these small bones are disappearing in man (Joseph, 1951).

Movements in the interphalangeal joint

During the grasping movement the distal phalanx of the thumb is extended or slightly flexed. The degree of flexion and extension is dependent on the shape and position of the object and on the relative length of the thumb. Wide individual differences are also seen in the flexion-extension excursion of the distal phalanx. According to Harris and Joseph (1949), in Europeans the maximal flexion angle varies from 24° to 92° and the extension angle from 0° to 67°. A limitation of movement in the interphalangeal joint is usually easily compensated for by movements in the joints of the other fingers. Even a complete loss of movement with retention of sufficient stability, as for instance in an arthrodesis, has no severe consequences for the power grip, but precision movements such as are required for writing, or the tying of shoelaces, are done awkwardly.

Stability of the interphalangeal joint in the lateral and axial directions is obtained by means of the collateral ligaments, stability in the dorso-volar direction by the long flexor and extensor of the thumb. In some functional movements of the thumb not belonging to the prehensile movements, the distal phalanx is maximally extended, for instance in pressing on a thumbtack. In these actions the extension is stabilized not by the flexor pollicis longus but by bilateral check-ligaments running from the volar plate of the distal phalanx to the ' osteo-fibrous tunnel of the proximal phalanx (Littler, 1960).

Function of the intrinsic muscles

The complex formed by the thenar muscles can be seen as a segment of a cone having as its vertex the base of the proximal phalanx (Fig. 3). Due to the radial position of the first metacarpal in this conic segment, the muscle mass on the ulnar side of the cone has, from the mechanical point of view, the most favourable position. This is in accordance with the function of the various muscles. The adductor pollicis primarily provides the thumb with grasping power. The radial muscle group, which consists of the abductor pollicis brevis, the opponens pollicis, and the superficial head of the flexor pollicis brevis, implements the grasping movement. The deep head of the flexor pollicis brevis occupies a transitional position, both anatomically and functionally (Tubiana and Valentin, 1968). By successive contractions of these partially overlapping muscles, a fluent swinging motion of the thumb is brought about, which is necessary for precision handling.

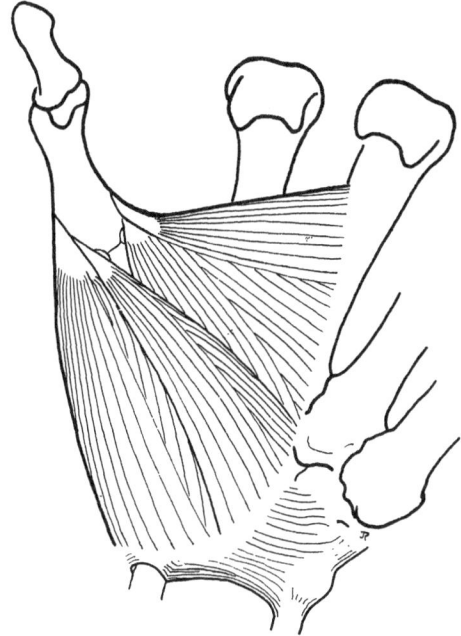

Fig. 3. The thenar muscles as segment of a cone.

The *abductor pollicis brevis* arises from the transverse volar carpal ligament and the radial carpal eminences. The muscle frequently receives additional slips arising from the tendon of the palmaris longus and the abductor pollicis longus. The muscle fibres run roughly parallel with the first metacarpal and are gradually grouped in two parts. The ulnar belly inserts on the radial side of the base of the proximal phalanx. A few fibres run along the border of the extensor apparatus to the distal phalanx. The radial, more superficially situated belly has a fan-shaped insertion on the tendon of the extensor pollicis longus (Napier, 1952). Von Lanz and Wachsmuth (1962) mention an insertion on the radial sesamoid. The abductor brevis brings the first metacarpal into abduction and a slight flexion, and the proximal phalanx into abduction and a small degree of pronation. At the same time, the abductor, by its expansion to the extensor apparatus, can play a contributory role in the extension of the distal phalanx (McFarlane, 1962; Kaplan, 1965). This muscle is responsible for the main part of the opposition movement: the departure of the thumb from the plane of the hand palm and its placement opposite the other fingers. It then makes it possible for the thumb to maintain contact with the distal phalanx of the index and middle fingers, these fingers being meanwhile extended in the inter-phalangeal joints and flexed in the metacarpo-phalangeal joints (Duchenne, 1867). This action is of especial importance for precision handling.

The *opponens pollicis* lies under the abductor brevis. Its fibres run in a dorso-radial direction to the radial aspect of the first metacarpal. Its function, which is the rotation and slight abduction and flexion of the first metacarpal, seems modest, but as the only rotator on the extreme radial side of the thenar muscle cone, this muscle is indispensable for precision handling. Forrest and Basmajian (1965) observed on electromyograms that at 'soft' opposition the opponens showed the greatest amount of activity of the three radial thenar muscles, while in 'firm' opposition the flexor pollicis dominated.

The *flexor pollicis brevis* is composed of a superficial and a deep head. The origin of the former is located slightly distal to that of the abductor brevis. It inserts on the radial sesamoid and radially on the base of the proximal phalanx. A few fibres extend into the extensor apparatus. The deep portion arises in the vicinity of the capitate bone and inserts on the radial and sometimes also on the ulnar sesamoid. Day and Napier (1961) assumed that the insertion of the deep head has phylogenetically undergone a shift from ulnar to radial. This shift, whether or not complete, they thought to be related to the acquisition of true opposability in Primates. The confusion in the literature concerning the deep head could be avoided, according to

Jones (1944), if the flexor brevis were considered as a muscle inserting only on the radial sesamoid. The muscle flexes, pronates, and abducts the first metacarpal and the proximal phalanx, and supports the extension of the distal phalanx. The flexor brevis can, without the help of the abductor brevis and the opponens, bring the pulp surface of the thumb into contact with the volar side of the middle phalanx of the other four fingers, even when the latter are flexed in the meta-carpo-phalangeal joint and extended in the interphalangeal joints (Duchenne, 1867). As compared to the abductor brevis, the flexor brevis can flex the first metacarpal further and has appreciably less abductive capacity, in the deeper portion even none at all.

The *adductor pollicis*, with its oblique and transverse heads, occupies the ulnar portion of the thenar cone. Coming from the third meta-carpal and from structures located around the base of the second metacarpal, the muscle fibres run partially perpendicular to the longitudinal axis of the thumb to the ulnar sesamoid and the ulnar aspect of the base of the proximal phalanx. The superficial insertion fibres spread out in the extensor apparatus. The adductor moves the first metacarpal in the direction of the second, and flexes the metacarpo-phalangeal joint. It also brings about an extension of the distal phalanx and a limited supination of the proximal phalanx. The stabilizing effect of the flexor brevis and the adductor on the metacarpo-phalangeal joint is of paramount importance for the power grip. According to Rabischong (1964), the flexor tendons of the index finger form a kind of retinacular apparatus with respect to the adductor when the thumb is in opposition.

The *first dorsal interosseous* arises from the first and second meta-carpals and inserts mainly on the base of the proximal phalanx of the index finger (Landsmeer, 1955). This muscle is able to adduct and supinate the thumb when the index finger is stabilized by other muscles.

Function of the extrinsic muscles

The *flexor pollicis longus* is primarily a flexor of the distal phalanx of the thumb. Only toward the end of the flexion movement in the interphalangeal joint does some flexion occur in the metacarpo-phalangeal joint. The long flexor has almost no influence on the carpo-metacarpal joint. This muscle is important in precision hand-ling. Flexion of the distal phalanx occurs in almost complete inde-pendence of flexion in the other fingers. The functional independence of the thumb flexor is a comparatively recent acquisition in the evolution of the hand, existing only in man (Mangini, 1960). And, after all, is not precision handling a typically human action? In the power grip the flexor pollicis longus serves chiefly as a stabilizer of the interphalangeal joint. The flexor longus makes a real contribution to the power of the grip only when the distal phalanx of the thumb as it were locks the grip by pressure exerted on the dorsal side of the fingers, as in the action of chopping with an axe.

The *extensor pollicis longus* – formerly called the extensor pollicis adducens – extends both the proximal and the distal phalanges of the thumb and brings the first metacarpal into extension, adduction, and limited supination. During the extension-adduction movement the tendon shifts, with respect to the base of the first metacarpal, about 5 mm in the ulnar direction. This muscle is involved in many aspects of the grasp function. Together with the extensor pollicis brevis and the abductor pollicis longus it effects the extension of the thumb in the opening of the hand. It contributes to the precision of the move-ment of the distal phalanx and the stabilization of the interphalangeal joint and, lastly, the retroposition of the thumb. The adductive action of the muscle acquires considerable compensatory value for the grasp function in cases of ulnar nerve paralysis (Mannerfelt, 1966).

The extensor pollicis longus is flanked at the level of the proximal phalanx by the abductor and adductor expansions (Fig. 4 on p. 32). Although the extensor apparatus of the thumb ends abruptly at the level of the base of the 'second' phalanx; it shows a strong resem-blance to the extensor apparatus of the fingers (Baumann, 1947).

The *extensor pollicis brevis* inserts dorsally on the base of the pro-ximal phalanx of the thumb. Usually, a few fibres become continuous with the extensor pollicis longus tendon. The muscle extends the metacarpo-phalangeal joint and brings the first metacarpal into extension and to a slight extent into abduction. It enables the thumb to remain extended in the metacarpo-phalangeal joint while the distal phalanx is flexed. This is important for precision movements such as the downstroke in writing. In this connection it is remarkable that the muscle only occurs completely separated from the abductor pollicis longus in man (Jones, 1944; Kaneff, 1968).

The *abductor pollicis longus* occurs in several variants. In 80 per cent of the cases one or two accessory tendons are present, having their insertion in the vicinity of the base of the first metacarpal. In about 30 per cent there is an insertion on the abductor pollicis brevis. At least one tendon always has an insertion on the radio-dorsal side of the base of the first metacarpal (Stein, 1951; Fenton and Lapidus, 1953; Schmidt et al., 1968). The muscle brings about an abduction-extension in the carpo-metacarpal joint. It also has a role in the opening of the hand and, together with the extensor pollicis brevis, supports the abductor pollicis brevis in the initiation of the opposition movement. In the power grip it is an indispensable stabilizer of the carpo-metacarpal joint, i.e. it prevents an outward sliding of the base of the first metacarpal radially when there is strong traction of the adductor pollicis.

The opposition of the thumb is supported by two extrinsic muscles that do not belong to the thumb musculature. During this movement, the *extensor carpi ulnaris* and the *palmaris longus* contract, as can easily be observed in most humans. The extensor carpi ulnaris neutralizes radial deviation in the wrist joint activated by the abductor pollicis longus. The role of the palmaris longus in opposition is less clear. That it tightens the transverse carpal ligament seems doubtful (Kaplan, 1965). If several insertion slips spread out in the fascia of the abductor brevis or the hypothenar, the part played by this muscle is clear, but in many cases these slips are not present. Conceivably, during opposition the palmaris longus neutralizes in its turn the extension of the wrist joint effected by extensor carpi ulnaris, thus serving as the last link in the chain of the opposition system.

The role of the hypothenar muscles – synergists of the thenar muscles – in the grasp function of the hand lies beyond the scope of the present study.

The power grip and precision handling have been indicated (page 4) as constituting the basic pattern of the grasping movements of the hand. The main characteristic of the power grip is the static phase, i.e. the rigid relationship between the hand and the object, the movement taking place in the wrist, elbow, and shoulder joints. This static phase is preceded by a dynamic phase consisting of the opening of the hand, the positioning of the fingers, and the approach of the fingers to the object (Landsmeer, 1962). If the object is so small that in approaching it the pulps of the distal phalanges of the thumb, index finger, and middle finger almost touch each other, one speaks of the pinch grip or pinch *(pincement, Spitzgriff)*. This constitutes a power grip in which the precision element is very pronounced and the need for power is secondary. In precision handling there is, in principle, no static phase.

Nerve supply of the intrinsic muscles

The innervation pattern of the thenar musculature shows numerous variations, from complete median nerve to complete ulnar nerve innervation (Murphey et al., 1946; Cliffton, 1948; Rowntree, 1949). The most frequent pattern is innervation of the abductor brevis, the opponens, and the superficial head of the flexor brevis by the median nerve, the ulnar nerve supplying the deep head of the flexor brevis, the adductor, and the first dorsal interosseous. In about 5 per cent of the cases the abductor brevis is additionally innervated by the ulnar nerve or the adductor by the median nerve. Innervation of the opponens by the ulnar nerve or of the first dorsal interosseous by the median nerve is seldom seen. Variations in the innervation of the flexor brevis occur frequently. In thirty dissections, Day and Napier (1961) found a dual nerve supply of the superficial head seven times and a dual nerve supply of the deep head of the muscle five times.

This pattern of innervation is furthermore frequently crossed by anastomoses, which occur in some cases between the median and ulnar nerves (Kaplan, 1965; Mannerfelt, 1966; Jones and Goldner, 1966). In the proximal part of the lower arm about 15 per cent show an anastomosis – called after Martin and Gruber, who first described it – comprising motor or sensory fibres or both. The motor fibres go to the adductor and first dorsal interosseous, among others. In the carpal region there is a median-ulnar shunt known as the Riche-Cannieu anastomosis. The nature of this latter connection and the frequency of its occurrence are still unknown.

The radial nerve may also be involved in the nerve supply of the thenar muscles. Many authors have described fine branches deriving from the superficial branch of this nerve and running to the abductor brevis, as reviewed by Grünkorn (1932) and Kaplan (1965).

CHAPTER II

FUNCTIONAL LOSS IN PARALYSIS OF INTRINSIC THUMB MUSCLES

Paralysis of radial thenar muscles

When the action of the abductor pollicis brevis, the opponens, and the superficial head of the flexor pollicis brevis is lost, the thumb can no longer be brought into opposition, which seriously impedes the grasp function of the hand. Only cylindrical objects of limited size can still be firmly grasped. Because of the absence of opposition of the thumb, precision handling is no longer possible.

When the action of the flexor pollicis brevis remains intact, coordination with the abductor pollicis longus makes an *incomplete opposition* possible. This means that with a limited abduction and pronation, the thumb can be placed opposite the fingers. The abduction of the thumb – measured as the diametral distance between the distal flexion crease of the thumb and the base of the extended middle finger – amounts to only 2 to 4 cm, as compared to the normal distance of 7 to 8 cm. Pronation is not only limited, but also occurs too late in the movement. In other words, when the thumb has already passed the index finger, a rather abrupt rotation of about 45° occurs. This pronation can be measured from the rotation of the thumbnail with respect to the palm of the hand, which in a normal opposition amounts to between 70° and 100°. Therefore, a spherical object can only be grasped in the hand if the diameter of the object is less than 4 cm and the fingers are extended in the metacarpophalangeal joints and flexed in the interphalangeal joints. The force of the grasp is also diminished, since the carpo-metacarpal joint is only stable when abduction (or adduction) is complete. Furthermore, the adductor cannot develop maximal power in an incomplete abduction, because 'a muscle can exert greater force when it is on a stretch than when it is shortened' (Wells, 1955). Precision handling is hampered because, as a result of the limited abduction, the thumb can only follow the fingers if their metacarpo-phalangeal joints remain extended and their interphalangeal joints flexed. Extension of the thumb is accompanied by some adduction of the first metacarpal, since the abductor brevis is no longer able to neutralize the adductive effect of the long extensor muscle of the thumb. As a consequence, movements requiring precision, such as writing, are performed rather spasmodically and awkwardly, with shortening of the excursive movement.

In paralysis of the median nerve, a normal opposition movement is possible only when there is an anomalous innervation, possibly combined with insertion of the palmaris longus into the fascia of the abductor brevis.

In cases of a high median nerve paralysis, the loss of thumb function is increased by a paralysis of the flexor pollicis longus.

Paralysis of ulnar thenar muscles

With paralysis of the ulnar nerve, the grasping force between the thumb and fingers is reduced to at least half the normal value (Björkesten, 1946; Bunnell, 1956; Matev, 1960). For a large part of this loss, the adductor paralysis is responsible. Mannerfelt (1966) found that after an ulnar nerve block the adductive force of the thumb was reduced to 20 per cent of the normal value. He also found that strength of the adduction in patients with a rupture of the extensor pollicis longus tendon dropped to nil after an ulnar nerve block. The adductive capacity of the extensor pollicis longus is well known, but some authors assign the same capacity to the flexor pollicis longus (v. Lanz and Wachsmuth, 1959; Bowden and Napier, 1961; McFarlane, 1962).

The compensating adductive effect of the extensor pollicis longus is accompanied by an often obstructive flexion of the distal plahanx. This flexion increases the greater the adductive force required (Froment's sign). This is probably not due to a reduced capacity for extension of the distal phalanx in consequence of the paralysis of the adductor or to a kind of claw mechanism analogous to that of the fingers, but rather to a strong compensatory contraction of the flexor pollicis longus, as a result of which the tension of the extensor pollicis longus is increased and the adductive force becomes more effective (Boyes, 1964).

In low ulnar nerve lesions the most important functional distur-bance is, according to Zrubecky (1960), the incomplete, claw-like, and weak pinch grip. The pinch grip is performed in a typical way, the most pronounced form occurring when the superficial head of the flexor brevis also does not function. When an attempt is made to press the pulps of the thumb and the index finger together with some force, the middle phalanx of the index finger shows marked flexion and the proximal phalanx shows extension, ulnar deviation, and supination. This ulnar deviation of the index finger in the pinch grip is produced by the adductive action of the extensor indicis proprius and the long flexors of the index finger. With paralysis of the first dorsal interosseous, this action dominates over the abductive action of the extensor digitorum communis of the index finger. The adduction of the meta-carpo-phalangeal joint of the index finger is linked to a supination (Landsmeer, 1955). The thumb is in the extension, adduction, and supination position and is hyperextended in the metacarpo-phalan-geal joint, to the extent that the ligaments of the joint permit. The distal phalanx of the thumb is markedly flexed. The extended distal phalanx of the index finger slides off in the proximal direction along the volar side of the thumb, as a result of which the thumb is still in contact with the radial side of the proximal phalanx of the index finger. All that is left of the pinch grip is a kind of key grip. With some effort, a small smooth object (such as a nail) can be picked up with this key grip if the upper arm is abducted and elevated and the lower arm pronated.

Precision handling is also no longer possible, not so much because of the anomalous movement of the thumb but because of the limited lateral and axial movements of the fingers, the clawing of the ring and little fingers which is often present, and the absence of the hypothenar elevation.

Paralysis of radial and ulnar thenar muscles

With paralysis of all the intrinsic thumb muscles, the disturbances seen in an isolated median or ulnar nerve paralysis occur in combination and are even enhanced (Fig. 9 and 22). Little remains of the thumb movements. The extensors of the thumb can still effect extension or adduction-extension of the first metacarpal, but in this movement the proximal phalanx is held in extension and the distal phalanx in flexion. The flexor pollicis longus can only flex the extended first metacarpal to the neutral position. Due to the loss of the opposition movement and the adductive force of the thumb, the anomalous flexion pattern of the fingers, which in flexing as it were curl up, the instability of all the metacarpo-phalangeal joints, the usually present clawing of the fingers, and the absence of the hypothenar elevation, hardly anything is left of the grasp function of the hand. If, in addition, the loss of sensibility of the entire volar side of the hand is taken into account, there can be said to be a physiological amputation of the hand (White, 1960). Nevertheless, a number of useful functions remain, such as the hook grip, for instance for carrying a handbag, and the interdigital squeeze. Between the index and middle fingers, the latter usually gives sufficient strength to hold a light object such as a pen, and between the proximal phalanx of the thumb and the distal part of the second metacarpal, this sideways pinch is of even more importance, since a certain degree of dexterity is sometimes attained with it that can be lost after tendon transfer.

These disturbances can become even more complicated, especially in combined paralysis of the median and ulnar nerves, if contracture develops. The flattening of the transverse metacarpal arch, the clawing of the fingers , and the hyperflexion of the distal phalanx of the thumb can easily acquire a fixed character. This is rapidly followed by an adduction (-extension) contracture of the thumb due to shrivelling of ' the skin, fascia, and muscle tissue in the first intermetacarpal space and of the capsule of the first carpo-metacarpal joint. The tendon of the extensor pollicis longus threatens to become luxated and fixed in the ulnar direction, and some cases show a chronic subluxation of the base of the first metacarpal radially.

Whereas in a distal ulnar nerve paralysis the loss of motor function is primary, in a distal median nerve paralysis the loss of sensibility predominates. Loss of sensibility on the volar side of the thumb and the index and middle fingers means, with respect to the already limited precision handling, that only inadequate information can be obtained concerning the amount of pressure applied, the position of the joints, and the position and shape of the object. The power grip, or what remains of it, becomes uncertain; often, more force is applied than is necessary. At the same time, trophic changes occur, most pronounced in median nerve paralysis. The limited capacity of the circulation of the hand to adapt to low temperatures can greatly increase the disability. The absence of tactile gnosis, or even of protective sensibility, however, does not mean that the hand is entirely useless (Moberg, 1966). The best evidence of this is provided by the results of tendon transfers in leprosy patients (Brand, 1966). A certain amount of compensation is provided by effective coordination with the sight and by training in the interpretation of pressure and stretch stimuli, which are observed, via transmission, in the marginal regions of the normally radial-nerve innervated skin.

Prognosis of median and ulnar nerve lesions

The recovery of sensibility and of intrinsic motor function after median and ulnar nerve suture is inadequate in more than one-third of the cases, although the prognosis is much more favourable for children. Recovery of sensibility is rated good for the median as well as the ulnar nerve in about 30 per cent of the distal lesions, but a two-point discrimination of less than 15 mm is seldom regained (normal 2 to 5 mm). In low median nerve lesions, recovery of motor function after 5 years is rated good in about 25 per cent of the cases; for low ulnar nerve lesions this figure is about 20 per cent (Zachary, 1954; Nicholson and Seddon, 1957; Flynn, 1962; Önne, 1962). The percentages of motor recovery are based on the recovery of muscular strength. The figures provide no information about the recovery of independent action, rapidity of contraction, amplitude, control of motion, and endurance (Moberg, 1968). The recovery of muscular strength does not necessarily mean recovery of function. Furthermore, the percentages would be appreciably lower if an abnormal innervation pattern were excluded pre-operatively for isolated nerve lesions. According to Moberg (1969), true recovery of the function of the thenar muscles almost never occurs.

Refined techniques of nerve repair, such as the funicular or selective-funicular nerve suture (Hakstian, 1968), cannot be successfully applied to the median nerve because of the complex intraneural topography. The funicular pattern of the ulnar nerve, on the other hand, makes it more suitable (Sunderland, 1968).

Palliative reconstruction of the volar sensibility of the thumb in isolated median nerve lesions can be done by means of a neurovascular skin island transfer taken from a region of the skin of the ring or little finger innervated by the ulnar (Littler, 1959; Hueston, 1967), or, if the ulnar nerve is also severed, from the dorsal side of the proximal phalanx of the index finger (Holevich, 1963). However, the beneficial effect of this operation is small in cases with a volar anaesthesia of the index and middle fingers. The protective sensibility is usually restored sufficiently to save the hand from frequent wounds.

Nevertheless, the palliative reconstruction of the function of the thenar muscles forms an indispensable component of the treatment of the paralytic hand, and this holds particularly for the opposition tendon transfer.

CHAPTER III

RECONSTRUCTION OF THE OPPOSITION

Indications

For a useful grasp function of the hand it must be possible for the thumb to be placed opposite the middle finger with an abduction distance (page 15) of at least 2.5 cm. In about 30 per cent of the isolated lesions of the median nerve this position is not reached, and an opposition reconstruction should be considered (Kirklin and Thomas, 1948). When such lesions are combined with a lesion of the ulnar nerve, this holds for almost 100 per cent of the cases. It must be kept in mind here that for a normal grasp function an abduction distance of at least 4 to 5 cm is necessary (Mangini, 1968).

In proximal nerve lesions such as a brachial plexus lesion or lesions of the spinal cord following a low cervical injury, reconstruction of the opposition is only worth considering when the excursion and force of the movements of the elbow, wrist, and finger joints have been adequately recovered (Luckey and McPherson, 1947; Lipscomb et al., 1958). Opposition reconstruction can also give improvement of the grasp function in selected cases of spastic paralysis (Goldner, 1955).

Other indications include a long-standing compression of the median nerve, e.g. in a carpal tunnel syndrome (Littler, 1967), disturbed opposition resulting from traumatic loss or aplasia of thenar muscles, poliomyelitis, and, in Eastern countries, especially due to leprosy. In cases of pollicization of a finger for reconstruction in amputation or hypoplasia of the thumb, it is not always possible to achieve adequate opposition of the new thumb (Huffstadt, 1960; Hage, 1966). In such cases the new thumb can be brought into the desired position by an opposition tendon transfer (Harrison, 1964; Edgerton et al., 1965).

In the evaluation of the indications, weight must be given to the age of the patient and the length of the interval between the injury to the nerve and the suture. In children the prognosis of a nerve suture is in general favourable, and as a rule a wait-and-see policy should be adopted with respect to a tendon transfer. But when, in a child, the recovery of opposition after a median nerve suture can no longer be expected, an opposition reconstruction should not be postponed: although it is often difficult to explain to children how they can bring their thumb into opposition after a tendon transfer operation, experience has shown that it is just in children that this operation can be performed successfully (Jacobs and Thompson, 1960). A maximum age cannot be stated; everything depends upon the physical and mental condition of the patient. In general, the results of tendon transfers in older patients are less satisfactory, partly because of the slow cortical reorientation with respect to the changed motor pattern.

How long one should wait after a median nerve suture before performing a reconstruction of the opposition, depends upon the expectations with respect to the recovery of the motor function. Some authors advise waiting for one or two years (Lange, 1953; Schink, 1962), others perform a tendon transfer at the same time as the nerve suture (Deyerle and Tucker, 1960). White (1960) suggests waiting three to four months before deciding, basing his decision on the evidence of motor return and, in high median nerve lesions, on the advancement of Hoffmann-Tinel's sign. If the reconstruction is postponed any longer than this, even intensive rehabilitation cannot entirely prevent the development of secondary deformities. In some cases, such as a self-inflicted injury to the wrist, prompt reconstruction of opposition and therefore a quick return to normal employment can be more important than the disadvantage of a retrospectively superfluous tendon transfer.

Prerequisites

Opposition tendon transfers are, like all tendon transfers, subject to a number of conditions, as stated by Mayer (1916), Bunnell (1956), and others. The most important prerequisite is that the thumb must be able to be brought into opposition passively. An opposition tendon transfer cannot overcome an adduction contracture of the thumb. If there is a limited contracture, an attempt can be made to abolish it by physiotherapy and a dynamic splint. When the adduction contracture has a fixed character, however, surgical correction is required. This correction consists of a skin plasty in the thumb web, the fascial structures of the first intermetacarpal space also being released. In some cases the insertion of the transverse head of the adductor must be cut and the first dorsal interosseous stripped from the first metacarpal, in combination with a capsulotomy of the first carpo-metacarpal joint and a tenolysis of the extensor pollicis longus tendon. In severe contracture at the base of the thumb, excision of the trapezium is sometimes performed (Tubiana and Lord, 1955; Goldner and Clippinger, 1959).

The extrinsic muscles of the thumb must function adequately. If these muscles function only partially or not at all, an opposition tendon transfer will fail because of instability of the thumb, overcorrection of the opposition, and atrophy of the transferred muscle. Under the most favourable circumstances, a tenodesis effect of the transferred tendon will persist.

The formation of adhesions must be limited. A small amount of adhesion over the entire length of the transferred tendon is unavoidable and even necessary for its vascularization. These fine adhesions permit a certain amount of excursion after a period of muscular activity. The portion of the mesotenon that is transferred together with the tendon regains its function to some extent (Smith and Conway, 1966; Colville et al., 1969). If the tissue in the immediate vicinity of the tendon is also movable with respect to the neighbouring structures, as is the case for the subcutis and paratenon tissue, an almost normal amplitude of tendon motion is guaranteed. Scar tissue and damaged periosteal and fascial structures must therefore be avoided as much as possible on the transfer route.

The transferred muscle must possess sufficient strength to surmount the traction of the antagonists and the resistance offered by the adhesions and the pulley mechanism.

The physiological length of the muscle must be maintained as correctly as possible by the application of the proper amount of tension. With too much tension, the muscle is overstretched; and too little tension reduces the amplitude of the muscle. Both too much and too little tension lead to atrophy of the muscle. It is impossible to determine precisely the amount of tension under which the transferred tendon must be sutured in place to obtain optimal function, but tetanic nerve stimulation after release of the tourniquet may supply useful information (Williams, 1965). In the literature, almost without exception, a tension which is slightly too high is preferred to one which is slightly too low. Brand (1966) advises that the thumb be brought to complete opposition while the wrist is kept in the neutral position, and that the tendon then be pulled about 1 cm from the slack position before it is stitched.

In tendon transfers the traction of the muscle-tendon unit should generally be as much as possible in a straight line. In opposition tendon transfers this rule is usually not held to, because the tendon must pull in a given direction to form an angle of about 45° with the longitudinal axis of the lower arm.

The integrity of the muscle should be maintained, so that it can provide one motion essential to function (Boyes, 1964). An accessory tendon of the abductor pollicis longus cannot be transferred for the reconstruction of the abduction-flexion movement of the first metacarpal while the actual abductor longus tendon continues to pull the thumb into abduction-extension. At the most, the inefficient resultant action of the two movements will be obtained.

The result of an opposition tendon transfer depends less on the method applied than on the extent to which the above-mentioned conditions can be satisfied (Kirklin and Thomas, 1948; Jacobs and Thompson, 1960).

Historical background

The principle underlying transfer of a tendon of an intact muscle to compensate for the loss of function of one or more paralytic muscles was first applied by Nicoladoni in 1882 in a case involving the lower leg. The earliest publications on tendon transfers in the arm for the treatment of paralysis of a radial nerve, which appeared in 1898, were soon followed by many papers on this subject. In 1911, Lange reported the experience accumulated in more than a thousand tendon transfers in the arm and leg, but made no mention of the treatment of a median nerve paralysis. Eight years later, Hass noted that the literature on irreparable median paralysis was extremely scarce; he mentioned two authors, one of whom, Spitzy, discussed loss of opposition of the thumb, which he proposed in 1918 be treated by an arthrodesis of the carpo-metacarpal joint. In the same year, Steindler made the first mention of a tendon transfer to obtain opposition, and he was soon followed by many others.

It is striking that the opposition tendon transfer developed relatively late; and the sudden marked increase in interest in the restoration of opposition is even more remarkable: by 1930, 15 publications had appeared, 12 of which concerned different methods. But although the literature on opposition reconstruction continued to accumulate, reconstruction of adduction of the thumb and abduction of the index finger took 24 years longer (Bunnell, 1942) to attract attention.

This irregular development of tendon transfers cannot be entirely explained by two World Wars, epidemics of poliomyelitis, and advances in tendon surgery. Van den Berg (1969), who has discussed the changing nature of matter and mind under the term metabletics, argues that scientific progress is related to the pattern of living characterizing a given period. The development of the opposition reconstruction, to the extent that it involves scientific innovation, would then have to be explained in terms of a metabletic background.

Methods

The objective of opposition reconstruction is to compensate for loss of the action of the radial thenar muscles by transfer of a muscle or tendon. In these cases the gain with respect to the grasp function must more than counterbalance the secondary dysfunction involved in the removal of a muscle or tendon. It is impossible to completely replace the complex structure of the radial thenar muscles by the transfer of one muscle or tendon. What can be achieved is the abduction and flexion of the first metacarpal, together with abduction and limited pronation of the proximal phalanx of the thumb. Pronation of the first metacarpal can also be obtained, but seldom more than partially.

Muscle transfers

The ideal motor to replace the action of the radial thenar muscles is the abductor of the little finger, since this abductor is a synergist with about the same amplitude as the abductor brevis of the thumb. The muscle has sufficient power for the restoration of opposition and can be transferred to the thumb without intervening pulley or gliding tendon. The weakened abduction of the little finger has relatively little importance for prehension. A certain amount of abduction will in any case remain possible due to the action of the extensor proprius and the flexor brevis of the little finger. It is hardly surprising that transposition of the abductor digiti quinti is one of the oldest methods for opposition reconstruction.

Huber and Nicolaysen both introduced the method in 1921, according to Nicolaysen (1922) independently. This elegant and effective method received no recognition in the literature until 1963 – thus all of 42 years later – when Littler and Cooley once again drew attention to it.* According to them, this method has two disadvantages: it offers technical difficulties and, like every neurovascular pedicle transfer, involves some risk. Furthermore, the ulnar nerve must of course be intact. The technique is as follows: both tendinous slips of insertion of the abductor digiti quinti are divided, the muscle is dissected free, and the proximally situated neurovascular pedicle is isolated. The origin of the muscle is also detached from the pisiform bone, only the connexion with the tendon of the flexor carpi ulnaris being retained. The muscle is then turned over like the page of a book and brought under the thenar skin, after which its tendons are sutured to the abductor brevis insertion.

Another, albeit less satisfactory, possibility for a muscle transfer to restore the opposition is the transfer of a portion of the adductor pollicis (De Vecchi, quoted by Littler, 1963).

Tendon transfers

Tendon-transfer methods for the restoration of opposition are difficult to classify, because most of them differ in the choice of the motor,

---

* According to van den Berg (1969), independent simultaneous improvements form one of the basic elements of metabletics. If the improvement is conceived, applied, and made known to the world too early, it is forgotten and only much later rediscovered.

the use of a fulcrum, the direction of pull of the transferred tendon, and the manner of insertion. The best classification is perhaps according to the motor used.

Almost all the flexors and extensors of the lower arm, whether or not lengthened with a tendon transplant, have been used and described as the motor for an opposition tendon transfer. It is understandable that for the first transfer of this kind an attempt was made to compensate for the functional loss of the intrinsic thumb muscles by transfer of the tendon of an extrinsic thumb muscle.

Transfer of the flexor pollicis longus tendon

Steindler (1918) split the distal portion of the flexor pollicis longus tendon into two parts, freed the radial half from its insertion and brought it around the radial side of the thumb, and then inserted it dorsally on the base of the proximal phalanx. The opening made in the tendon sheath of the long thumb flexor served as fulcrum or, as it is usually termed, pulley. This was the first dynamic method to be devised for reconstruction of opposition, and was to be applied by many surgeons, as it still is. The method is simple and the secondary functional loss limited, but the abduction effect is small.

Howell (1926) cut the tendon of the flexor pollicis longus at the wrist, drew the distal end out of its sheath, and led it around the ulnar side of the thumb across the extensor pollicis longus tendon and then subcutaneously over the thenar and the transverse carpal ligament, re-attaching it at the wrist to the proximal part of the tendon. The opening in the antebrachial fascia functioned as pulley.

Silfverskiöld (1928) severed the flexor pollicis longus tendon at the level of the metacarpo-phalangeal joint of the thumb. The proximal part was led around the radial side of the thumb and inserted on the first metacarpal, and with the distal end a tenodesis of the interphalangeal and metacarpo-phalangeal joint was performed.

Von Baeyer (1932) lifted the tendon out of its sheath by means of a large longitudinal incision in the thumb, leaving the tendon intact. The tendon was then looped over the tip of the thumb and, via a circular incision around the thumb, brought under the skin.

Makin (1967) modified von Baeyer's method by 'translocating' the

flexor pollicis longus tendon dorsally via an osteotomy of the proximal phalanx of the thumb.

Williams (1966) frees the flexor pollicis longus from its insertion,
draws it via an incision near the wrist from its sheath, and leads it
first under the transverse carpal ligament and then subcutaneously
over the thenar to the proximal and distal phalanges of the thumb.

Transfer of the abductor pollicis longus tendon

Scherb (1945) detached the abductor pollicis longus tendon from its
insertion and re-inserted it at a point more ulnar and distal to the
original insertion on the first metacarpal.

Edgerton and Brand (1965) also use the abductor pollicis longus.
The tendon is brought over the brachioradialis around the radial side
of the wrist, drawn under the palmaris longus tendon as pulley,
and then, subcutaneously, back to the base of the first metacarpal,
after which it is sutured in place slightly distal to the original insertion.
In this way the tendon remains superficial to the antebrachial fascia.
This method is combined with an adduction tendon transfer.

Transfer of the extensor pollicis brevis tendon

Zancolli (1965, 1968) in complicated cases transfers the extensor
pollicis brevis tendon under the radial artery in a radial direction
and then via the radial portion of the carpal tunnel to the proximal
phalanx of the thumb. This requires passing through the antebrachial
fascia.

Transfer of an extensor tendon of a finger

Extensors of the fingers were also used very early for the restoration
of opposition.

Cook (cited by Taylor, 1921) drew one of the extensor tendons of
the little finger around the ulnar side of the wrist and then subcutaneously over the thenar to the first metacarpal.

Jahn (1929) did the same with the extensor of the middle finger.
The extensor defect was repaired with a free fascial transplant.

Zancolli (1965, 1968) also sometimes uses the extensor indicis proprius, which is led via the ulnar side of the wrist to the proximal phalanx of the thumb.

Price (1968) passes the extensor indicis proprius between radius and ulna in the volar direction and then around the palmaris longus tendon, as pulley, to the thumb. This transfer is combined with a transfer of the superficial flexor tendon of the middle finger.

Transfer of the tendon of a wrist extensor

It was rather late in the development of opposition reconstruction that a wrist extensor was chosen as motor.

Phalen and Miller (1947), in cases in which flexors were not suitable for transfer, used the extensor carpi ulnaris as motor. The tendon was led around the ulnar side of the wrist and, after being lengthened with a tendon transplant, was brought subcutaneously to the thumb.

Iselin (1955) did the same, but drew the tendon under the palmar fascia, the radial edge of the fascia serving as pulley.

Henderson (1962) obtained good results in such cases by transfer of the extensor carpi radialis longus or brevis around the ulnar side of the wrist. He also used the brachioradialis.

White (1962) even preferentially chose one of the wrist extensors as motor.

Transfer of the palmaris longus tendon

Ney (1921) used the palmaris longus, mainly because of its limited functional importance. The tendon of this muscle, which runs through the most superficial part of the antebrachial fascia, was led under the fascia. As extension he used the tendon of the extensor pollicis brevis, which he cut at the level of the wrist joint, drew under the transverse carpal ligament, and sutured to the palmaris longus tendon. In the absence of the palmaris longus he used the flexor carpi radialis as motor, the transverse carpal ligament serving as pulley.

Camitz (1929) inserted the tendon of the palmaris longus, lengthened with a strip of the palmar fascia, on the radial side of the metacarpophalangeal joint of the thumb. In this method a pulley was not used, the tendon passing along the volar side of the transverse carpal ligament.

Transfer of a flexor digitorum superficialis tendon

Krukenberg (1921) split the flexor superficialis tendon of the middle finger in two and inserted the radial half at the site of the insertion of the opponens*.

Bunnell mentioned the method of Camitz as early as 1924, but found that better results were obtained if the flexor superficialis of the ring finger was drawn through a pulley construction in the vicinity of the pisiform bone and then subcutaneously to the distal end of the first metacarpal. Later (1938), he inserted the tendon dorso-ulnarly on the base of the proximal phalanx. As alternative motor he used the flexor carpi ulnaris lengthened with a tendon graft. The pulley construction consisted of a loop with a diameter of 2 cm, made of a free tendon graft and attached to the origin of the abductor of the little finger. Another possibility was to split the tendon of the flexor carpi ulnaris and turn one half over in the distal direction to attach it to the pisiform bone. Also, the palmaris longus tendon could be cut 4 cm proximal to its insertion and the distal end of the tendon fixed to the pisiform bone. Lastly, instead of a loop construction, the transferred tendon could be led around the ulnar side of the flexor carpi ulnaris tendon. This last procedure has the advantage that the paratenon of the wrist flexor provides for ample gliding of the transferred tendon and, in addition, the method is less complicated. To bring the superficialis tendon into a subcutaneous position, it must pass through the antebrachial fascia. The edge of the opening made in the antebrachial fascia keeps the transferred tendon in place to some extent during the opposition movement, and this prevents a marked change in the direction of pull. This method devised by Bunnell, i.e. the transfer of a superficialis tendon of the ring finger to the thumb via a pulley situated near the pisiform bone, was rapidly accepted by many surgeons as a safe, effective, and relatively simple way to restore opposition, most of them preferring the flexor carpi ulnaris as pulley. Many modifications of this method have been published.

* This method has a metabletic aspect. Transfer of an entire superficialis tendon would have been less harmful for the function of the middle finger, technically somewhat simpler, and, with respect to the restoration of opposition, more effective. A man as ingenious as Krukenberg must have considered this, but in 1921 the cutting of half of a superficialis tendon was quite progressive enough.

Roeren (cited by Kochs, 1932) brought the superficialis tendon of the ring finger through an opening in the distal part of the transverse carpal ligament and from there to the first metacarpal.

Kiaer (cited by Bohr, 1953) did the same via an opening in the proximal part of the ligament.

Royle (1938) led the superficialis tendon of the ring finger through almost the entire length of the sheath of the flexor pollicis longus. An important element of his method was that he attached one slip of the tendon to the insertion of the flexor pollicis brevis and the other dorsally on the first metacarpal.

Thompson (1942) drew the superficialis tendon of the ring finger distal to the transverse carpal ligament in a volar direction and from there around the ulnar edge of the palmar fascia, as pulley, to reach the thumb subcutaneously. One slip of the tendon was fixed distally to the first metacarpal, the other dorso-ulnarly to the base of the proximal phalanx.

Littler (1949) preferred an attachment of the superficialis tendon on the abductor brevis insertion. With respect to the pulley, Littler later (1960) made a distinction between an isolated paralysis of the median nerve and a combined median and ulnar nerve paralysis. In the former the flexor carpi ulnaris tendon was used as pulley, but in the latter the radial distal margin of the transverse carpal ligament was taken for this purpose so that the transferred tendon would pull in a direction intermediate between opposition and adduction.

Riordan (cited by Jacobs and Thompson, 1960) modified Littler's mode of insertion by suturing the tendon both to the abductor brevis insertion and to the tendon of the extensor pollicis longus at the level of the proximal phalanx of the thumb.

Brand (1966) uses two insertion slips for cases of paralysis of both the median and ulnar nerves. One is led across the neck of the meta-carpal, superficial to the extensor tendons, and sutured to the insertion of the adductor pollicis. The other is brought along the radial aspect of the metacarpo-phalangeal joint volar to the flexion-extension axis and then, just proximal to the interphalangeal joint, attached to the extensor pollicis longus tendon under a slightly higher tension than the first slip. In this way not only does one tendon slip run on the volar and the other on the dorsal side of the flexion-extension axis but at the same time one is situated on the radial and the other on the ulnar side of the abduction-adduction axis (Fig. 4). The intention of this opposition tendon transfer is therefore to achieve an extension of the distal phalanx, stabilization of the meta-carpo-phalangeal joint, and abduction, flexion, and rotation of the first metacarpal. This, however, does not simplify the mode of insertion. For the pulley, Brand also made use of the naturally fibrous tunnel of Guyon, which lies just to the radial side of the pisiform bone.*

Palazzi (1962) pointed out another possible pulley in the vicinity of

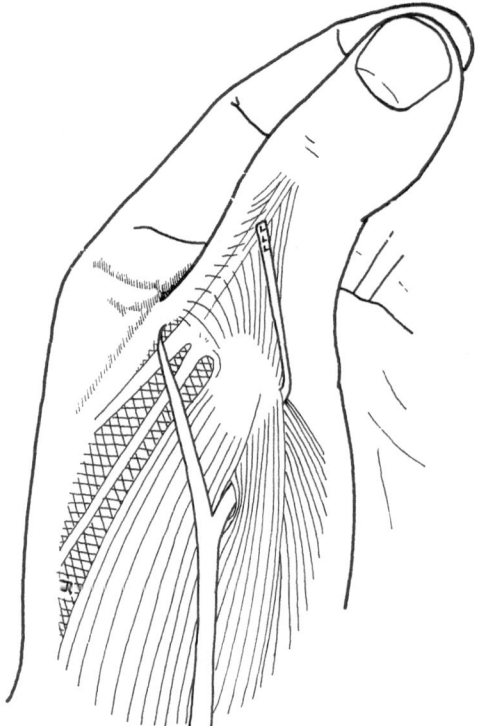

Fig. 4. Insertion of opposition tendon transfer after Brand.

* The ulnar artery and nerve reach the hand via this triangular tunnel, which is bordered on the ulnar side by the pisiform bone, on the dorsal side by the transverse carpal ligament, and volarly by the thickened antebrachial fascia, reinforced by an expansion of the flexor carpi ulnaris tendon.

the pisiform bone. He drew the superficialis tendon under the origin of the abductor of the little finger, using the pisiform bone as fulcrum. Göbell and Freudenberg (1935) transferred the proximal half of the superficialis tendon of the little finger to the thumb, the remaining distal portion of the tendon being sutured to the superficialis tendon of the ring finger.

Transfer of a flexor digitorum profundus tendon

Jacobs and Thompson (1960) reported obtaining good results with a transfer of the profundus tendon of the little finger in which, in analogy with the method of Göbell and Freudenberg, the remaining distal portion of the profundus tendon was sutured to the profundus tendon of the ring finger.

The insertion

In the description of the various methods for tendon transfer it is striking to note that initially the insertion was made on the first metacarpal, whereas later the tendon was attached radially or dorso-ulnarly to the base of the proximal phalanx. The objection to a single insertion on the proximal phalanx of the thumb is that with even a slight shift the transferred tendon comes to lie either on the volar side of the flexion-extension axis of the metacarpo-phalangeal joint, which causes hyperflexion of the proximal phalanx, or on the dorsal side of this axis, as a result of which there is a tendency to hyperextension of the proximal phalanx. Such a slight shift of the tendon can occur readily if the metacarpo-phalangeal joint has a wide flexion-extension range. Once a hyperflexion of the proximal phalanx has occurred, the flexed thumb will work as a lever arm in the pinch grip and, as a result of the pressure of the index and middle fingers, the first metacarpal will be rotated into supination. This shifting of the tendon at the metacarpo-phalangeal joint can be prevented if the tendon is attached to the insertion of the abductor brevis. Although this mode of insertion does not provide either flexion or pronation of the proximal phalanx, it is nevertheless the ideal insertion in cases with paralysis of the radial thenar muscles.

This can be easily understood if it is kept in mind that a complex movement like opposition cannot be completely realized by a single tendon transfer and that it is chiefly the action of the abductor brevis which must then be compensated for.

Another way to prevent shifting of the tendon is the double insertion. It is far from easy, however, to achieve the correct tension on both tendon slips, especially since the tension ratio of the slips changes during opposition. In cases of median and ulnar nerve paralysis, if one tendon slip is sutured to the abductor brevis insertion and the other to the tendon of the extensor pollicis longus, a good position of the proximal phalanx will be obtained initially and at the same time the frequently present hyperflexion of the distal phalanx will be corrected. But since there is no adductor action, the chance is great that eventually the ligaments on the ulnar side of the metacarpo-phalangeal joint will be stretched by the traction of the transferred tendon and the pressure of the fingers during the grasping movement. As a result, there will be hyperabduction of the proximal phalanx of the thumb. In cases of paralysis of all the intrinsic thumb muscles, therefore, the ingenious double insertion devised by Brand is the most suitable method. This double insertion stabilizes the metacarpo-phalangeal joint, prevents a secondary hyperabduction deformity of the proximal phalanx, and corrects the hyperflexion of the distal phalanx.

In the method of Edgerton and Brand the insertion angle of the abductor longus tendon, i.e. the angle formed by the tendon with the longitudinal axis of the first metacarpal, is increased, as compared to its original size, by the transfer via the palmaris longus tendon. This means that the angulating moment of the muscle has been increased and its stabilizing power decreased. Consequently, this method is only suitable for cases in which the adductor action has been lost, and a less powerful stabilizer of the carpo-metacarpal joint is required. In combination with an adduction tendon transfer the method gives the thumb adequate stability.

If the metacarpo-phalangeal joint of the thumb is stabilized by the ulnar thenar muscles or by a capsulo-plasty, an adduction tendon transfer, or an arthrodesis, each transferred motor-tendon unit can in principle be attached proximally to the first metacarpal. The more proximally the insertion is made, the smaller the lever arm of the muscle. This has the consequence that a greater muscular force and a smaller amplitude are required to achieve the same position of opposition, because work equals force times distance. Therefore, when only a powerful muscle with a limited amplitude is available for an opposition tendon transfer, this muscle should be inserted proximal to the first metacarpal, to make the most efficient use of power and amplitude. One of the disadvantages of this insertion is that in paralysis of the median and ulnar nerves provision must also be made for the stability of the metacarpo-phalangeal joint.

If necessary, the lever arm can also be made larger and at the same time the abductive action of the muscle can be increased by introducing (after Le Coeur, 1953) a bone graft about 1 cm thick between the transferred tendon and the base of the first metacarpal.

The pulley

If a tendon transfer is intended to compensate for loss of action of the radial thenar muscles, the direction of pull of the transferred tendon must be roughly parallel to the direction taken by the fibres of these muscles, i.e. in a direction running from the metacarpo-phalangeal joint of the thumb to a point in the vicinity of the pisiform bone. If traction is exerted in this direction, the first metacarpal moves in abduction and flexion. If an extensor of the wrist or a finger is transferred around the ulnar side of the wrist and then passed sub-cutaneously to the thumb, the tendon acquires the correct direction almost automatically. The edge of the ulna then functions as fulcrum. To avoid disturbing the gliding of the tendon over this fulcrum, the anastomosis between the wrist extensor and the free tendon graft must be made proximal to the fulcrum, i.e. dorsally on the lower arm. But if a flexor tendon is transferred, a fixed point must be found in the wrist region to serve as fulcrum, preferentially where adhesions to this point can be expected to be very limited. Such adhesions can be expected to form more readily in a constructed pulley than in a natural one. The direction of pull of the tendon is determined by the location of the pulley. If a semicircle is drawn on the palm of the hand and the wrist, with as its centre the carpo-metacarpal joint of the thumb and as diameter the distance from this joint to the

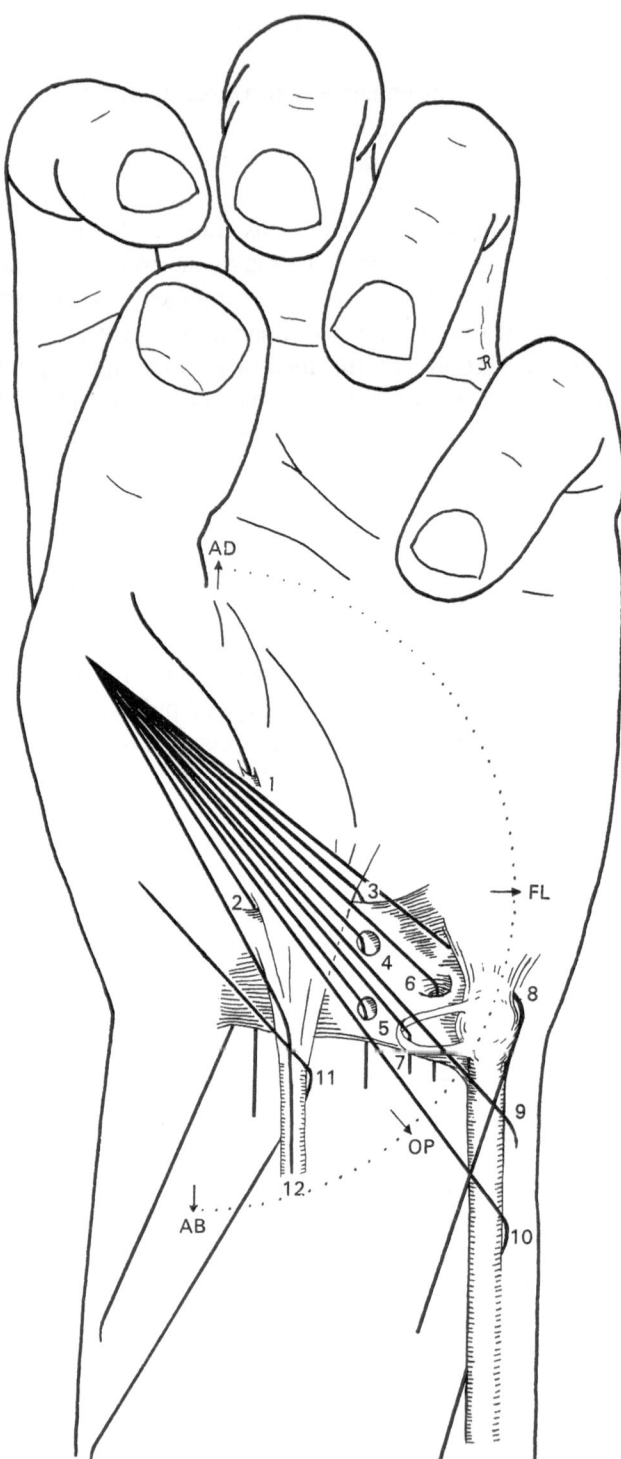

Fig. 5. Various possibilities for a pulley mechanism.

pisiform bone, the pulley possibilities within this semicircle can be shown schematically as in Fig. 5. These possibilities are:

1. Margin of the opening in the tendon sheath of the flexor pollicis longus. Steindler (motor: flexor pollicis longus).
2. Distal margin of transverse carpal ligament. Ney (motor: palmaris longus); Littler, in median and ulnar paralysis (motor: sublimis IV); Williams (motor: flexor pollicis longus); Zancolli (motor: extensor pollicis brevis).
3. Ulnar margin of the palmar fascia. Thompson (motor: sublimis IV).
4. Window distally in transverse carpal ligament. Roeren (motor: sublimis IV).
5. Window proximally in transverse carpal ligament. Kiaer (motor: sublimis IV).
6. Guyon's tunnel. Brand (motor: sublimis IV).
7. Sling at pisiform bone. Bunnell (motor: sublimis IV).
8. Pisiform bone. Palazzi (motor: sublimis IV).
9. Ulnar margin of ulna. Phalen and Miller, Henderson (motor: wrist extensor); Cook (motor: extensor V); Zancolli (motor: extensor II).
10. Ulnar margin of flexor carpi ulnaris tendon. Bunnell (motor: sublimis IV).
11. Ulnar margin of palmaris longus tendon. Edgerton and Brand (motor: abductor pollicis longus).
12. No pulley. Camitz (motor: palmaris longus).

The line of pull running roughly parallel to the fibre direction of the abductor brevis, cuts the semicircle at the point OP. If it cuts the semicircle at a point situated more proximally or radially, the abduction component will increase and the flexion component decrease. At the point AB the flexion component is reduced to zero; but distally, the flexion increases at the expense of the abduction. At the point FL, abduction is reduced to zero. If the line passes through the point AD, only adduction will occur. It is therefore possible, depending upon whether more abduction or more flexion is desired, to choose a proximal or a more distally situated pulley. In the total absence of opposition, as in a median and ulnar nerve paralysis, the line of pull should cut the arc in the vicinity of the point OP. When there is incomplete opposition, i.e. an opposition in which the abduction limitation predominates, the line will have to pass through a point situated between OP and AB. The most distally situated pulley is the one used in Steindler's method. The abduction component is small in this case. In Camitz's method, which does not make use of a pulley, at the neutral position of the wrist joint a pure abduction of the first metacarpal is obtained. With an ulnar deviation of the hand, the direction of the palmaris longus tendon runs parallel with that of the abductor brevis fibres and a flexion component is added.

Pressure or friction at the site of the pulley leads to a loss of effective power, the loss being greater the shorter the angle at which the tendon is bent. This angle is most acute with the method of Edgerton and Brand.

The motor

For the choice of the most suitable motor for an opposition tendon transfer, several factors must be taken into account:

1. Which muscle-tendon units are still active and show little or no damage, so that they might be suitable for transfer?
2. Which of these muscle-tendon units are transferable without giving a secondary dysfunction that would be as severe or worse than the dysfunction of opposition?
3. What is the relationship between power and amplitude in these muscles?
4. Which of these muscles are synergists to the thenar muscles?
5. Which muscle-tendon units have given good restoration of opposition empirically?
6. Where is scar tissue located?
7. Will muscle-tendon units be required for other tendon transfers as well?

These factors will be discussed in the same sequence.

1. *Availability:* Which muscle-tendon units are still active and have undergone little or no damage will depend upon the nature, extent, and localization of the injury and the result of the primary treatment.

It is not always easy to determine whether a given muscle functions normally, but an electrical investigation can contribute useful information.

2. *Dispensability:* The extent to which a muscle can be dispensed with for prehension is dependent on the degree to which synergists can take over its function. This functional non-essentiality is greatest for the palmaris longus, a muscle which is absent without functional limitation in 15 per cent of the cases. The flexor carpi radialis can be considered dispensable if the extensor carpi radialis longus (and abductor pollicis longus) can effect the radial abduction of the hand and the flexor carpi ulnaris guarantees flexion of the wrist. As early as 1922, Starr pointed to the importance of retaining one powerful wrist flexor in tendon transfers. Preferentially, this must be the flexor carpi ulnaris, because the most important movements in the wrist joint are the ulnar flexion and the radial extension. The power of the flexor carpi ulnaris, furthermore, is about twice that of one extensor carpi radialis muscle.

At least one of the wrist extensors should also be retained, preferentially one of the two carpi radialis extensors. Although the extensor carpi radialis longus and brevis have roughly the same power and amplitude, the effective extension power of the brevis is greater due to its insertion at the apex of the carpal arch, where it has the greatest lever arm with respect to the radio-carpal flexion-extension axis (Littler, 1960). Therefore, with transfer of the extensor carpi radialis longus there is less reduction of the wrist extension. Of the three wrist extensors, the extensor carpi ulnaris is the most suitable for an opposition tendon transfer as far as both functional non-essentiality and location are concerned.

Transfer of the extensor digiti proprius tendon of the index or little finger means that these fingers can no longer be extended individually, but this is not a serious impediment. In cases of paralysis of the median and ulnar nerves, the adductive action of the extensor indicis proprius can be intensively exploited by the patient for the interdigital squeeze between the index and middle fingers. The common muscle belly shared by the extensor digitorum communis tendons makes these tendons unsuitable for an opposition transfer, as will be discussed in detail below. The extensor pollicis brevis plays an important role in precision handling. Precision handling cannot be completely restored by a tendon transfer in cases of median nerve paralysis, and is further limited by transfer of the extensor brevis. The routine use of the tendon as an extension of, for instance, a wrist extensor, is therefore incorrect. The muscle can be used as a motor if other, less essential, muscles are not available. The extensor pollicis longus is essential for the functioning of the thumb.

The abductor longus is essential – quite apart from its function in the opening of the hand and in opposition – for the stabilization of the first carpo-metacarpal joint. Transfer of the tendon may therefore only be applied in cases with paralysis of the adductor pollicis, and then only on condition that the stabilizing function of the muscle is preserved to some extent, i.e. that after transfer the tendon is attached in the vicinity of its original insertion.

With the transfer of the flexor sublimis tendon of the ring, middle, or little finger, the secondary loss of function is usually small, but sometimes there is an objectionable loss of function in the donor finger. The removal of a superficialis tendon has the consequence that the flexion power of the finger is reduced and the flexion-extension balance of the finger is disturbed, which changes the flexion pattern. In that case the flexion power of the profundus tendon is only effective for the middle phalanx when the tendon has already flexed the distal phalanx, whereas normally the flexion begins simultaneously in both the distal joints. If the intrinsic muscles of the finger are intact, at flexion of the distal phalanx there will be a tendency to extension of the middle phalanx, because the extensors of the proximal interphalangeal joint, which remain active during the flexion movement, no longer have a dominating antagonist. If this tendency of the middle phalanx to extend cannot be inhibited by tense ligaments of the proximal interphalangeal joint, the middle phalanx will be deadlocked in hyperextension, and for a moment the finger will show the swan-neck deformity. The more the finger is bent in the meta-carpo-phalangeal joint, the less the power of the extensors of the proximal interphalangeal joint, until, with a kind of trigger effect, the middle phalanx suddenly snaps into flexion. Because of this finger imbalance and the reduction of the flexion power, White (1962) prefers to take a wrist extensor rather than a flexor superficialis as motor. In paralysis of the intrinsic finger muscles this recurvation tendency of the middle phalanx after removal of the flexor superficialis tendon does not occur. Transfer of a superficialis tendon is therefore likely to have a favourable effect on the clawing of the finger. In a high ulnar nerve lesion, with paralysis of the flexor profundus of the little finger – and usually of the ring finger, and in some cases of the middle finger as well – transfer of the flexor superficialis tendon is of course contra-indicated.

The flexor profundus can only be considered non-essential if the distal interphalangeal joint is stabilized due to ankylosis or by tenodesis or arthrodesis. But even in these cases, transfer of the flexor profundus of the index finger is inadvisable because of the great loss of power in grasping.

The flexor pollicis longus tendon is in principle not suitable for transfer unless the flexion of the distal phalanx can be maintained as well as a small amount of flexion of the proximal phalanx. The latter is important for the stability in cases with paralysis of all the intrinsic muscles of the thumb.

The pronator teres may be considered for an opposition tendon transfer when there is a median nerve lesion at the level of the middle of the lower arm in which the action of the pronator teres has survived. The muscle must be lengthened with a long tendon graft, e.g. the tendon of the plantaris longus.

The brachioradialis is a powerful stabilizer and flexor of the elbow joint, and consequently transfer of this muscle means a rather large loss of function for the arm.

3. *Power and amplitude:* In the choice of a motor for an opposition tendon transfer the power and amplitude of the muscles of the lower arm also play a part. The absolute power of a muscle is proportional to the number of fibres in a physiological cross-section, which cannot be accurately determined in pennate muscles. The power of a muscle is estimated to be 4 kg per cm^2 physiological cross-section (Hettinger, 1961). Even if it were possible to determine exactly the absolute power of the muscles of the lower arm, including that of the thenar muscles, it would still be impossible to say which muscles are the most suitable, with respect to power, for an opposition tendon transfer, since this is dependent on a number of factors which are

almost impossible to measure. These factors include the loss of effective power at the site of the pulley, the resistance encountered by the tendon due to adhesions, the resistance offered by a residual adduction contracture, the resistance of the antagonists, the influence of the direction of pull and of the manner of insertion on the ratio between the angulating, rotating, and stabilizing power of the muscle, and lastly, the distribution of the effective power over the various joints affected by the transferred muscle. It may be important, however, to know something about the mutual power relationships of the muscles of the lower arm. An impression of these relationsnips can be obtained from Table 1, taken from von Lanz and Wachsmuth (1959).

Table 1. Work capacity of the forearm muscles (in Mkg)

For flexion in the wrist joint:	
flexor digitorum superficialis	4.8
flexor digitorum profundus	4.5
flexor carpi ulnaris	2.0
flexor pollicis longus	1.2
flexor carpi radialis	0.8
abductor pollicis longus	0.1
abductor pollicis longus with radial deviation in wrist joint	0.4
palmaris longus	—
For extension in the wrist joint:	
extensor digitorum communis	1.7
extensor carpi ulnaris	1.1
extensor carpi radialis longus	1.1
extensor carpi radialis brevis	0.9
extensor indicis	0.5
extensor pollicis longus	0.1
For flexion in the elbow joint:	
brachioradialis	1.9
pronator teres	1.2
palmaris longus	0.1

The power of the palmaris longus is dependent on the development of its muscle belly, which varies widely. Because of this variability and the inconstant presence of its tendon, this muscle is in principle only suitable as a motor for tendon transfer if investigation shows clearly that it is capable of powerful contraction.

If a muscle with little power is chosen as motor, it may prove inadequate for the restoration of opposition in certain cases. For instance, when there is a limited mobility of the first metacarpal or heavy scarring along the transfer route, a powerful motor must be chosen preferentially. On the other hand, transfer of a powerful motor usually means a rather substantial secondary loss of function. In general, however, the power of the muscle is not decisive for the choice of the motor, because the amount of power needed for the opposition movement is relatively small.

The amplitude of the muscle seems to be of more importance for the choice of a suitable motor. The excursion required for a transferred tendon to bring the thumb from adduction-extension into opposition can be determined in a simple way. During opposition reconstructions the present author has found that in adults, with the wrist in neutral position, an excursion of about 3 cm is required if the flexor carpi ulnaris tendon is used as pulley and the abductor brevis insertion as point of insertion. For Camitz's method, in which no pulley is used, the necessary excursion is 2 cm; and for the method of Edgerton and Brand, in which the palmaris longus tendon is taken as pulley and the base of the first metacarpal as insertion, 1 cm excursion is needed. Because of the interference caused by adhesions, the excursion of the transferred tendon must in principle be greater than the values indicated above. Most of the muscles of the lower arm have an amplitude of more than 3 cm. Table 2 shows the total excursion of the various tendons of the lower arm, as given by Bunnell (1956), as well as additional data taken from Kaplan (1965).

Table 2. Total excursion of tendons in the forearm (in cm)

flexor digitorum profundus	II : 5	III : 8.5	IV : 7.6	V : 7.0
flexor digitorum superficialis	II : 5.3	III : 8.8	IV : 6.5	V : 6.0
extensor communis and proprius	II : 5.4	III : 5.5	IV : 5.5	V : 3.5
extensor pollicis longus	5.8			
flexor pollicis longus	5.2			
flexor carpi radialis	4.0			
extensor carpi radialis longus	3.7			
extensor carpi radialis brevis	3.7			
flexor carpi ulnaris	3.3			
extensor pollicis brevis	2.8			
abductor pollicis longus	2.8			
extensor carpi ulnaris	2.5			

According to Kaplan (1965), who found roughly the same excursion values:

brachioradialis	4.0
pronator teres	3.0

For tendon transfers a distinction is made between an absolute or actual and a relative or effective amplitude of the muscle (Boyes, 1962). The absolute amplitude is the distance over which a muscle can shorten maximally from a completely relaxed state, and is determined by the length of the muscle fibres. If the extensor carpi ulnaris, which has a limited absolute amplitude, is transferred via the ulnar side of the wrist to the thumb, inadequate opposition can occur when the wrist is in the neutral position. If the wrist is slightly extended, the transferred muscle becomes stretched and some shortening of the muscle can occur again, sufficient for a complete opposition of the thumb. The bi-articular wrist extensor has become a multi-articular muscle. The effective amplitude of the muscle is therefore increased by a movement of the intercalated wrist segment. If necessary, the required amplitude can be reduced by insertion of the tendon proximal to the first metacarpal, as in Edgerton and Brand's method. It may be stated that in general the amplitude of a muscle is not decisive for the choice of a suitable motor for the restoration of opposition. One of the advantages of a motor with a large amplitude is that for transference the tension on the muscle-tendon unit is less critical and can therefore be less exact.

4. *Synergism:* Many authors are of the opinion that the use of a synergist as motor for a tendon transfer is important for an optimal cortical coordination of the modified system of motion. In the opposition movement, the synergists are: the wrist extensors, of which the extensor carpi ulnaris plays the largest role in opposition, the palmaris longus, the flexors of the fingers and thumb, and the hypothenar muscles. According to Scherb (1945), it makes little difference, at least in the arm, whether synergists are used or not, because of the absence of '*antagonistischen Bindungen*' in movement of the upper extremity. Boyes (1964) also made no distinction for tendon transfers between synergists and antagonists. It proved possible to successfully transfer a wrist extensor for the restoration of the flexion of a finger, but also for the extension of a finger. Even a flexor digitorum superficialis could effectively extend a finger after transfer. An exception must be made here for the extensor digitorum communis: if a tendon of this muscle is transferred for the reconstruction of opposition, the thumb can be brought into opposition, but in grasping, because of the common muscle belly of the extensor, the opposition movement remains antagonistic, i.e. while the thumb goes into opposition the fingers are extended. For the flexor digitorum profundus, which also shares a common muscle belly, this does not hold, since it is a synergist to the thenar muscles.

5. *Empirical findings:* To select the most suitable motor for the reconstruction of opposition, it can be useful to know what muscles have been reported in the literature to give the best results. The number of publications on a series of opposition tendon transfers in which different muscles were used as motor and in which an analysis of the results of the various methods is given, is not large. Moreover, these series cannot be mutually compared, because of great differences in the nature of the opposition loss, the indications applied, the criteria used for the classification good-moderate-poor, the duration of the follow-up, and the average age of the patients, not to mention

differences in the way in which a given method was applied.

Nielsen (1946) obtained better results in 19 cases of poliomyelitis with Silfverskiöld's method (page 27) than with Ney's method (page 29).

Kirklin and Thomas (1948) compared for 75 cases of war injuries the results obtained with the use of the palmaris longus, the flexor and extensor carpi ulnaris, and the flexor superficialis IV as motor. They also compared the results with the pulleys of Thompson (Fig. 5, no. 3) and Bunnell (Fig. 5, no. 10). The best results were seen in cases in which the superficialis IV was transferred according to Bunnell, although good results were also obtained with the other motors. Of all the cases, the results in 44 per cent were classified as excellent and in 17 per cent as unsatisfactory.

Jacobs and Thompson (1960) gave a compilation of the results of 103 opposition reconstructions done mainly in poliomyelitis cases. As motor they used the flexor superficialis III and IV, flexor profundus IV and V, flexor carpi ulnaris, and palmaris longus. The Steindler method (page 27) was also applied. Of the total number of cases, 74 per cent were classified as good and 16 per cent as poor. Here, too, the results with the use of a flexor superficialis as motor were slightly better than those obtained with other motors. There was no difference between the results with the flexor superficialis III or IV.

Carayon et al. (1962) compared the results of Bunnell's method (Fig. 5, no. 10) with those of Steindler's method (Fig. 5, no. 1) in 30 cases of leprosy. Good results were obtained in 50 per cent of the cases and poor results in 10 per cent. There was little difference between the results of these two methods, but the criteria used for classifying the results included not only the pinching of the thumb with the index and middle finger but also pinching with the ring and little finger. For the latter, flexion rather than abduction of the first metacarpal is required, which would bias the evaluation of results obtained with the Steindler method.

It may be stated that the superficialis III and IV proved empirically to be suitable as motors, but that good or reasonably good opposition results can also be obtained with other muscle-tendon units.

6. *Presence of scar tissue:* An important factor in the choice of a suitable motor as well as of a pulley is the presence of scar tissue.

For example, when there is an extensive wound on the volar side of the wrist preference should be given to a wrist extensor as motor for an opposition tendon transfer over the transfer of a damaged flexor superficialis tendon, for which, moreover, a pulley construction is required. If the nature of the lesion makes it necessary to use a finger or wrist flexor as motor, the pulley can if necessary be kept out of the scarred region by choosing a more distally or more radially situated point as fulcrum. This procedure, however, does not provide optimal abduction-flexion of the first metacarpal. If the direction of pull is nevertheless to come from the vicinity of the pisiform bone and there is extensive scar tissue on the transfer route, the scarred region can be excised and replaced by healthier and more pliable tissue by means of a pedicle flap, and this may be the only available solution in cases with very severe scars. When the scarring is less severe another, simpler method can be applied more appropriately, i.e. the use of a *silastic* rod.

The principle and application of a pseudosheath, i.e. a mesothelial-like membrane of connective tissue that forms around a tubular foreign body, were tested in tendon surgery as early as 1936 by Mayer and Ransohoff. When the implantation material was removed after a few weeks and a tendon was introduced into the preformed channel, the vascularization of this pseudosheath proved adequate to supply the tendon graft, and the adhesions that developed between the tendon and the wall of the pseudosheath had a sufficiently fine structure to permit adequate gliding of the tendon. Milgram (1960) seems to have been the first to use a pseudosheath in opposition tendon transfers. As foreign material he used a strip of tantalum. But the application of the pseudosheath in tendon surgery only became practicable after the completely inert and also flexible silicone rubber proved to be an effective implantation material (Bassett and Carrol, 1963). Since then, the silastic-rod implantation has occupied an important place in the treatment of certain flexor tendon lesions. In Rotterdam, the silastic-rod implantation has been used successfully in cases with appropriate indications since 1965 (van der Meulen). Encouraged by the favourable results in flexor tendon lesions, we have also applied the silastic rod in opposition tendon transfers. The introduction of the silastic rod can be per-formed simultaneously with the correction of an adduction contracture of the thumb. To prevent retraction, the rod is fixed distally near the metacarpo-phalangeal joint of the thumb and can then be led subcutaneously to the tendon of the flexor carpi ulnaris or, if this muscle no longer functions, drawn through a window in the proximal part of the transverse carpal ligament, the window later being used as a pulley. After two months, the implant is removed and an opposition tendon transfer is performed, at which if necessary a silastic rod can again be introduced through the third intermeta-carpal cleft to the dorsal side of the hand so that a pseudosheath can be formed for a subsequent adduction tendon transfer for the thumb.

7. *Multiple motors:* Lastly, for the choice of a suitable motor for the reconstruction of opposition it is necessary to take into account the question of what other tendon transfers will have to be performed. For a high lesion of the median and ulnar nerves, an opposition tendon transfer will seldom be indicated. In a combined median and radial nerve paralysis, too, the functional loss is so great that the thumb can preferably be fixed in opposition. In an isolated high median nerve lesion, a motor should be available for the reconstruction of opposition, for flexion of the distal phalanx of the thumb, and also for flexion of the index and middle fingers. For this last, the flexor profundus tendon of the ring and little fingers is usually attached to that of the index and middle fingers.

Problems are offered by distal median and ulnar nerve lesions for which several tendon transfers are indicated even though in some cases a large number of muscles and tendons are damaged. If abduction of the index finger is to be restored, the tendon of the extensor indicis proprius and occasionally that of the extensor pollicis brevis can be transferred. Recovery of the adductive power of the thumb by a tendon transfer is only indicated when the patient's occupation demands powerful adduction of the thumb. In principle, this transfer requires a strong motor, preferably a flexor superficialis. For a dynamic correction of claw hand, an extensor proprius, a flexor superficialis, or a wrist extensor can be used. The treatment can be limited to a dynamic correction for the index and middle fingers, and for the ring and little fingers a capsuloplasty of the metacarpo-phalangeal joint (Zancolli, 1968).

Thus, the factor of other indicated tendon transfers must be taken into account in the choice of a motor for opposition reconstruction, but the latter is generally of such primary importance that it will be given preference when several motors must be chosen for various combined reconstructions.

Opposition by means of arthrodesis or tenodesis

If, due to the extent of the injury or paralysis, no suitable motor can be found for an opposition tendon transfer, the thumb can be fixed in the opposition position by an arthrodesis or a tenodesis.

To bring the thumb into opposition to the fingers in cases of paralysis of the median nerve, Spitzy (1919) performed an arthrodesis of the first carpo-metacarpal joint. With this method there is a considerable chance that the resulting opposition of the thumb, which still retains a small amount of mobility in the joint between the trapezium and scaphoid, will eventually be partially lost due to the traction of the opposition antagonists. A method providing greater stability is the introduction of a bone graft bridging the first and second metacarpals (Foerster, 1930; Thompson, 1942; Brooks, 1949). Both methods have the great disadvantage that with certain movements of the arm the thumb, which usually has only limited sensibility and always projects some distance out from the hand, is easily wounded. Furthermore, in this static opposition the compensatory adductive power of the extensor pollicis longus is eliminated, and in cases in which the radial nerve is still intact use cannot be made of the sensibility of the sides of the thumb and fingers. In some cases a troublesome hyperabduction develops in the metacarpophalangeal joint of the thumb, and an arthrodesis must also be performed in this joint. Consequently, great caution must be exercised in the application of these methods. They can even rob the patient of the last remnant of a serviceable hand function to which he may have already adjusted himself. It must be taken into consideration that in intermetacarpal arthrodeses Goldner and Irwin (1950) saw better recovery of function when a pseudoarthrosis had developed than when rigid union had been established between the first and second metacarpals.

A less static method is the opposition tenodesis, usually called opponodesis, in which a tendon graft is attached to the thumb at the level of the metacarpo-phalangeal joint, in principle in the same way as for the insertion of an opposition tendon transfer. If necessary, the tendon of the extensor pollicis brevis can be used for this purpose. The proximal end of the tendon is brought subcutaneously across the thenar, drawn through a drill hole in the distal end of the ulna, and then attached to itself. Both the distal and the proximal attachments to the bone must be very solid, since in a tenodesis there is no elastic system and, at least in the tenodesis itself, there are no receptors to signal the sudden occurrence of strong tension. The advantage of an opponodesis is that the degree of opposition can to some extent be regulated by active movements in the wrist joint. When the wrist is flexed the thumb can still be brought into the plane of the palm of the hand. Therefore, this method deserves preference over arthrodesis. The objection raised to the opponodesis or any form of tenodesis is that the fixed tendon may stretch (White, 1960), but if the indication for an opponodesis has been correctly evaluated, the forces that might be responsible for such stretching, such as those exerted by the wrist extensors, are usually limited. This remains true quite apart from the question of whether a tendon graft can indeed stretch. According to Brooks (1966), the most that can happen is that a teno-desis can become partially detached at its attachment on the bone, or rather on the periosteum of the bone, as a result of which the tendon could become slightly longer.

Supplementary corrections

If the hyperflexion of the distal phalanx of the thumb is not corrected by the opposition tendon transfer, this phalanx can be brought into its functional position by an arthrodesis. The functional position of the interphalangeal joint involves a flexion of about 20°, but in cases with severe pulp atrophy the distal phalanx should be fixed in exten-sion. If it is impossible to bring the distal phalanx into extension during the operation to reconstruct the opposition, the arthrodesis can be performed at the same time as the opposition tendon transfer.

When the metacarpo-phalangeal joint is found to have too little stability after the reconstruction of the opposition or remains in hyperextension or hyperabduction, correction can be effected by a capsuloplasty or an adduction tendon transfer. The most solid stabilization is obtained by an arthrodesis of this joint in a position with about 20° flexion, 15° pronation, and 10° abduction. This method is relatively simple and usually gives effective and lasting results.

CHAPTER IV

DISCUSSION OF SELECTED OPPOSITION RECONSTRUCTIONS

It will be clear from the preceding chapter that it is not possible to indicate which method of reconstruction is most suitable for a given case of opposition loss. The various aspects of the opposition reconstruction can, however, be illustrated by the discussion of a number of selected cases.

Case 1

History: This 16 year old patient was a compositor whose right hand was caught in a printing press. The badly swollen hand showed an oblique fracture of the third and fourth metacarpals, without displacement, and a skin wound on the radio-volar side of the wrist. In the field of the wound the median nerve and radial flexor tendons were undamaged. The fractures were immobilized by a plaster splint. After removal of the cast the middle and ring fingers were found to be in the claw position and the thumb could not be brought into opposition. The fractures had united in a satisfactory position, and it was hoped that a spontaneous recovery of the lost function would occur. We first saw the patient a year after the accident. He was unable to resume work because he could not pick up small letters. This precision handling requires good opposition but only limited adductive power of the thumb. A detailed analysis of the functional loss was made.

Examination: The radial thenar muscles showed atrophy. There was little filling of the second and third intermetacarpal spaces. The volume of the adductor muscle was distinctly smaller on the right than on the left. The appearance of the hypothenar was normal. The middle and ring fingers were slightly clawed. Although part of the flexor pollicis brevis was visibly and palpably tensed when an attempt was made to bring the thumb into opposition, the flexion of the first metacarpal was minimal and the pronation of the thumb amounted to only about 10° (Fig. 6). The maximal (abduction) distance between the radial surface of the thumb at the level of the distal flexion crease and the base of the index finger amounted to 2 cm. The adductive power of the thumb was limited. The pinch power between the thumb and the index finger, as measured with the Vigorimeter*, was half that of the left hand. The stability of the thumb was adequate in this situation, i.e. the joint was not hyperextended during the pinching action. The passive mobility of the thumb was normal. The sidewards movements of the middle and ring fingers were limited. The abduction of the little finger and the elevation of the hypothenar were normal. Remarkably enough, the sensibility was not disturbed. The patient had no paresthesia or aching discomfort, even when manual pressure was applied on the transverse carpal ligament. The ninhydrin finger-printing and the two-point discrimination tests did not reveal any anomalies.

Thus, there was an incomplete paralysis of intrinsic muscles as the result of a compression trauma, the function of the hypothenar muscles remaining completely intact. The findings were confirmed by the electromyographic investigation. The motor distal latency of the median nerve was somewhat prolonged (4.5 msec.), that of the ulnar nerve was normal. A lesion affecting a few of the motor branches of both these nerves in the region of the palm of the hand seemed probable. An exploration of this region, possibly with suturing of the motor branches, was considered. Because a year had elapsed since the accident, the chance of recovery of the motor function was small. It was decided to perform a reconstruction to restore the lost function.

Reconstruction: This was an ideal case for an opposition reconstruction: an actively cooperating young patient, no scars along the

---

* The Vigorimeter consists of a rubber bulb connected to a manometer. The bulb comes in three sizes (Fig. 11). With this apparatus a good impression can be easily obtained of the loss of grasp function of the hand or of the pinching power between the thumb and, for instance, the index finger, especially if the resulting values are compared with those obtained for the normal hand.

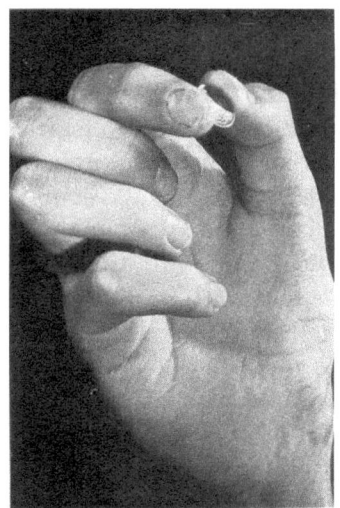

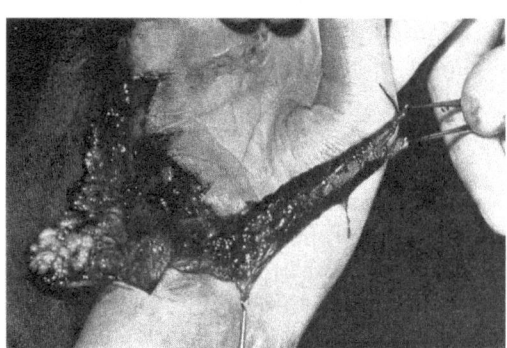

Fig. 7

Fig. 6

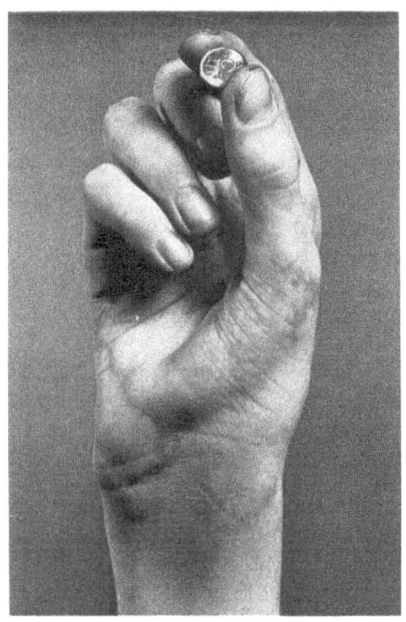

Fig. 6. Loss of opposition in an incomplete paralysis of intrinsic muscles.

Fig. 7. Restoration of opposition by abductor digiti quinti transfer.

Fig. 8. Result of the reconstruction.

Fig. 8

transfer route, normal passive mobility of the thumb with adequate stability in the metacarpo-phalangeal joint, and no restriction in the choice of a motor. It made little difference whether a superficial finger flexor, a wrist extensor, or the abductor digiti quinti was taken as motor. Since recovery of the opposition, or rather of the capacity for precision handling, was of primary importance for this patient, and the action of the radial thenar muscle can be compensated for most effectively by an intrinsic muscle participating in opposition, preference was given in this case to the reconstruction according to Huber and Nicolaysen. The abductor of the little finger was transferred to the thenar, where its two tendinous slips of insertion were sutured to the insertion of the abductor pollicis brevis (Fig. 7). A few weeks before the muscle transfer, the slight clawing of the middle and ring fingers was corrected by a capsuloplasty of the metacarpo-phalangeal joints.

Results: Upon removal of the bandage three weeks after the operation the patient was immediately able to bring his thumb into opposition and retroposition, although opposition was not complete. A month later he could bring the distal phalanx of the thumb opposite the base of the middle finger with an abduction distance of 6 cm (Fig. 8), the total pronation of the thumb amounting to 70°. The flexion of the first metacarpal was now normal. The patient was able to go back to work.

Case 2

History: This 21 year old patient was a carpenter who had fallen and cut his left wrist on a piece of broken glass. Exploration of the wound showed that the median nerve was completely severed, the ulnar nerve partially. The injury to the tendons was remarkably limited; only the palmaris longus was totally severed, the flexor superficialis tendon of the index finger subtotally. The nerves were repaired by primary suture.

Examination: Seven months after the nerve repair, the hand function was evaluated. The thenar was flattened and the intermetacarpal spaces had become deeper. Distinct atrophy of the hypothenar muscles was present only on the ulnar side (abductor digiti quinti). The scars in the wrist region felt supple. The thumb was in adduction-extension, and could not be brought actively into opposition. There was no sign of an adduction contracture, mainly because of the patient's very active cooperation in rehabilitation. The pinch power between the left thumb and index finger was one-third that of the right hand. During pinching the distal phalanx of the thumb was sharply flexed and the proximal phalanx extended (Fig. 9); the index finger deviated in the ulnar direction and showed supination. When an attempt was made to pinch as powerfully as possible, the index finger slid off the distal phalanx of the thumb. The patient could extend his fingers completely, and they showed no tendency to claw. The elevation of the hypothenar was good, the abduction of the little finger limited. Sensibility was restricted on the volar side of the hand, but the protective sensibility was adequate.

Reconstruction: This too was a favourable case for an opposition reconstruction, since there was little scarring in the wrist region and normal mobility of the thumb. There was no reason to consider transfer of the abductor digiti quinti in this case. The possibilities for a tendon transfer were not limited, but it was important that the pull be exerted in the right direction, so that both abduction and flexion of the first metacarpal would be obtained. In addition, the insertion of the transferred tendon had to be such that the stability of the meta-carpo-phalangeal joint of the thumb would be restored and the tendency of the distal phalanx to hyperflexion corrected. Because of the injury to the palmaris longus, transfer of the abductor longus tendon via the palmaris longus tendon was not suitable for this case. On the basis of functional dispensability, power, and amplitude, a transfer of the extensor carpi ulnaris tendon or of the flexor superficialis tendon of the ring finger deserved preference, and the latter was chosen.

The flexor superficialis tendon was cut at the base of the ring finger, drawn outward at the wrist, led around the flexor carpi ulnaris tendon, and then brought subcutaneously to the metacarpophalangeal joint of the thumb, where it was attached by the double-insertion method according to Brand. Two months later the abduction of the index finger was restored by detaching the extensor indicis proprius tendon at its insertion, drawing it under the tendon of the extensor pollicis longus, and then suturing it to the bony insertion of the first dorsal interosseous. The extensor indicis tendon was drawn under the tendon of the extensor pollicis longus to increase the adductive power of the long thumb extensor and to have the line of pull of the extensor indicis correspond as much as possible to the direction of the muscle fibres of the first dorsal interosseous. For the time being, an adduction tendon transfer was not indicated, especially since the patient was righthanded.

Results: The recovery of opposition was partially incomplete and partially overcorrected. The pronation of the thumb was 60° (*versus* 90° in the right hand). The maximal abduction distance between the distal flexion crease of the thumb and the base of the middle finger amounted to 9 cm, 1 cm more than on the right (Fig. 10). The flexion of the first metacarpal was adequate. The stability of the metacarpo-phalangeal joint was good. At strong pinching the hyperflexion of the distal phalanx was appreciably reduced. The adductive power of the thumb was slightly increased. The pinch power between thumb and index finger now amounted to about half that of the right hand, possibly achieved by the more advantageous angle of approach of the extensor pollicis longus tendon but also possibly because of training of the muscle. The abductive power of the index finger was sufficient to prevent ulnar deviation in powerful pinching (Fig. 11). The ring finger showed no tendency to recurvation at flexion. The

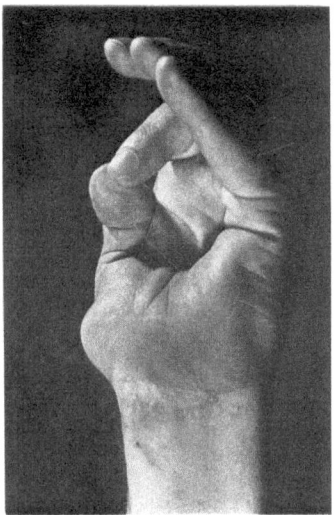

Fig. 9

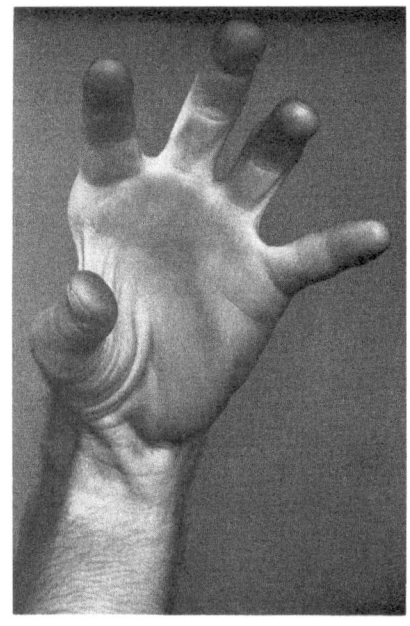

Fig. 10

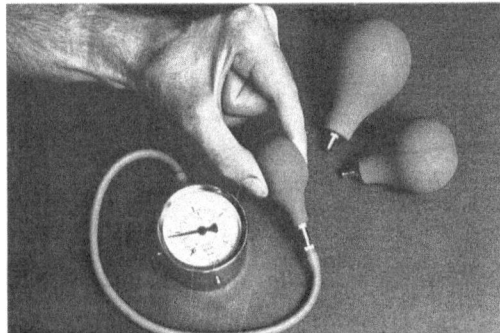

Fig. 11

Fig. 9. Pinch in a median and ulnar nerve lesion.

Fig. 10. Opposition restored by tendon transfer. Motor: sublimis IV; Pulley: flexor carpi ulnaris tendon.

Fig. 11. Vigorimeter for measuring the power of grasp and pinch.

patient was able to resume his work as a carpenter. Although he was generally satisfied with the functioning of the hand, he had one serious complaint. This concerned not the loss of power or sensibility but the discomfort and inconvenience arising from the fact that his left hand often became cold when he had to work outdoors.

Case 3

History: This patient, a 33 year old electrician, had attempted suicide by striking his right wrist with great force against a knife held between his feet. All the flexor tendons had been severed except the profundus tendon of the ring and little fingers. The median nerve, radial artery, thumb extensors, and both radial carpal extensors had also been cut through. The knife had driven deep into the wrist joint, but had done little damage to the bone structure (Fig. 12). At the time, the wrist joint was closed and the nerve and all the severed tendons were sutured. Although it is not usual to perform a primary nerve suture in such a serious wound, it was done in this case of a psychotic patient for whom the additional psychic pressure of the loss of the use of the hand had to be abolished as rapidly as possible. Postponement of reparative and reconstructive treatment would have increased the chance of another suicide attempt.

Examination: Three months after the injury the recovery of function was evaluated. The radial thenar muscles showed atrophy. The thumb could not be brought actively into opposition (Fig. 13). The adductive power of the thumb and the stability of the metacarpo-phalangeal joint were normal. Flexion of the distal phalanx of the thumb reached 90°, and there was no limitation of the extension. Individual flexion of the fingers was possible to a limited extent. The power of extension in the wrist joint was weak, abduction in the radial direction limited. The electromyogram of the radial thenar muscles showed scanty electric activity of a few motor units at voluntary effort. Although recovery of the motor function was possible it seemed unlikely to occur, and therefore surgical treatment was not postponed.

Reconstruction: Before choosing a suitable motor for opposition, the dorsal side of the wrist was explored. The continuity of both radial carpal extensors was partially intact, but there was little tension on the tendons and many adhesions had developed in the vicinity. The tendon suture had evidently not held at this point, and the defect was bridged by scar tissue. The tendons were resutured. Transfer of the extensor carpi ulnaris seemed to involve risks, and consequently the volar side was explored. The appearance of the median nerve was rather good; there was little thickening at the site of the suture and there were only fine adhesions to the surrounding tissue. The flexor superficialis tendon of the ring finger also showed little scarring at the site of the anastomosis, and this muscle seemed to offer a reliable motor for the reconstruction of opposition. To avoid the scar tissue in the superficial part of the wrist region as much as possible, a window in the proximal ulnar part of the transverse carpal ligament was taken as pulley. Some paratenon tissue of a neighbouring flexor tendon was drawn over the edge of the window to promote smooth movement of the transferred tendon over the pulley. The tendon was attached to the insertion of the abductor brevis.

Results: Recovery of opposition was not complete, but was nevertheless adequate (Fig. 14). The pronation of the thumb was 40°, the flexion of the first metacarpal a little too small. The maximal (abduction) distance between the distal flexion crease of the thumb and the base of the index finger was 6 cm. It seems possible that better results might have been obtained if a silastic rod had been implanted a few weeks before the tendon transfer. Retroposition was normal. The stability of the wrist was distinctly improved. Five months after the injury, the patient was able to make a vase in the occupational therapy department and give it a painted decoration with considerable precision. During the observation period in the psychiatric department, he worked as an electrician for the maintenance department of the hospital. The function of the hand would have permitted normal employment, but admission to a psychiatric institution proved necessary.

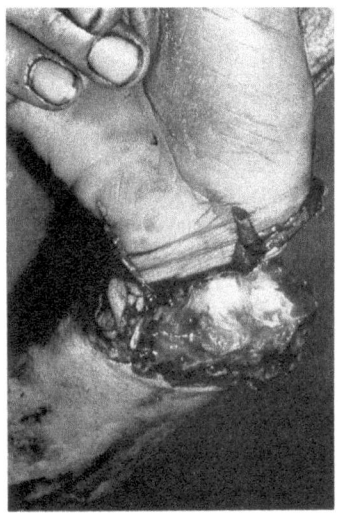

Fig. 12

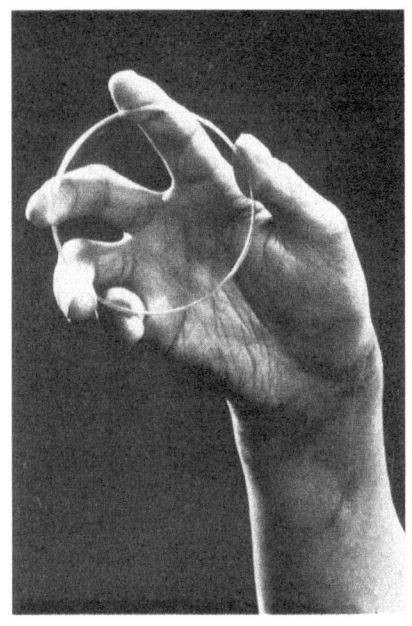

Fig. 13

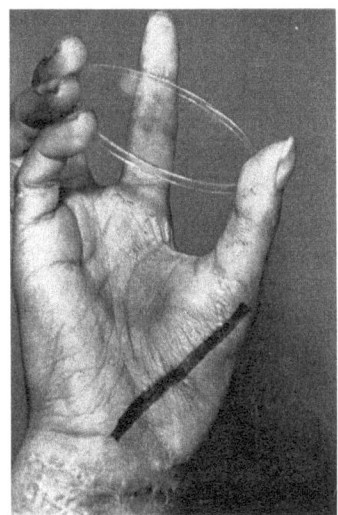

Fig. 14

Fig. 12. Self-inflicted injury to the wrist.

Fig. 13. Paralysis of radial thenar muscles.

Fig. 14. Adequate opposition after tendon transfer.
Motor: sublimis IV; Pulley: window in proximal ulnar part of transverse carpal ligament.

Case 4

History: A 23 year old sewing teacher had cut the volar side of her left wrist with a bread knife in a suicide attempt. Exploration of the wound showed that the median and ulnar nerves, the radial and ulnar arteries, and all the flexor tendons had been severed. All the tendons, both nerves, and the radial artery were sutured. The patient was admitted to the psychiatric department. The psychiatric prognosis was considered favourable, especially if the patient could return to her work with as little delay as possible.

Examination: Three months after the injury, all the intrinsic muscles showed atrophy. The thumb was in adduction-extension (Fig. 15); the distal phalanx showed hyperflexion, but could be extended passively. Active opposition was not possible. The strength of pinch between the index finger and thumb was one-fourth that of the right side. The fingers were slightly clawed and could be rolled up in the palm of the hand. The patient had paresthesia on the entire volar side of the hand.

Reconstruction: A motor was required for the restoration of the opposition of the thumb and for the correction of the claw deformity of the fingers. Because of the relatively recent anastomoses in the volar part of the wrist, a finger or wrist flexor did not seem suitable. The extensor carpi ulnaris was chosen as motor for the opposition reconstruction. The tendon of this muscle was lengthened with a free tendon graft, and then led around the ulna and drawn sub-' cutaneously over the thenar to the metacarpo-phalangeal joint of the thumb, where it was inserted according to Brand. The extensor carpi radialis longus was taken as motor for the correction of the claw deformity. To the tendon of this muscle were attached four free tendon grafts which were drawn separately in the volar direction through the interosseous spaces and then brought volar to the transverse metacarpal ligaments toward the lateral bands of the extensor apparatus. The insertion was located on the ulnar side of the index finger and the radial side of the middle, ring, and little fingers. This operation has been described by Brand (1961).

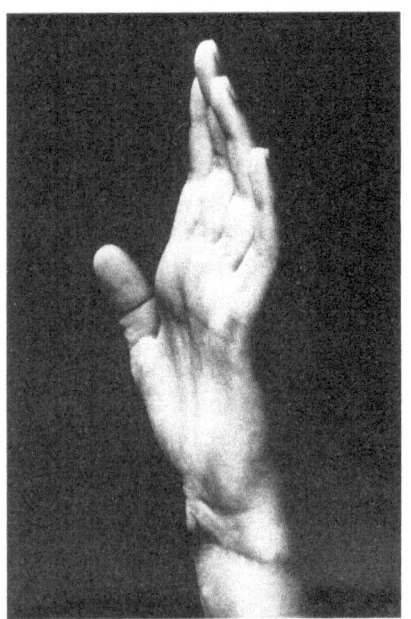

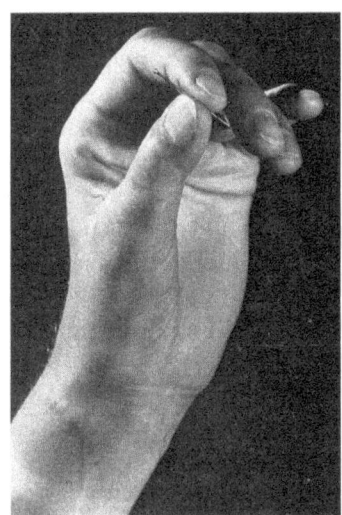

Fig. 16

Fig. 15

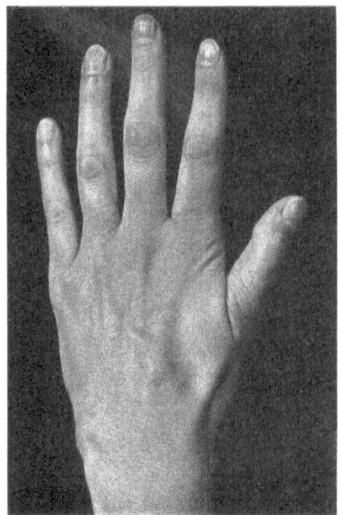

Fig. 17

Fig. 15. Paralysis of all the intrinsic muscles (enlargement of a frame from a 16 mm motion-picture).

Fig. 16. Opposition after transfer of the extensor carpi ulnaris tendon around the ulna.

Fig. 17. Correction of claw deformity by transfer of the extensor carpi radialis longus tendon.

Results: The recovery of opposition was good, although not ideal. The head of the first metacarpal could be placed opposite the shaft of the second metacarpal. The abduction distance between the distal flexion crease of the thumb and the base of the index finger at extension of the wrist was 6 cm. The thumb could only be pronated 20°. With this opposition tendon transfer, the hyperflexion of the distal phalanx was inadequately corrected, and two months later an arthrodesis was performed to stabilize the distal phalanx in a slightly flexed position (Fig. 16). Seen retrospectively, it would have been better to establish some pronation at the same time. The claw deformity of the fingers was almost completely corrected, and the patient could flex and extend her fingers virtually normally (Fig. 17). Eight months after the injury she resumed teaching. She complained only of the scars on the left hand, wrist, and foot (donor site of the tendon grafts). At examination two years after the injury, only the short flexor of the little finger could contract powerfully and there was insufficient re-innervation of the other intrinsic muscles, which was confirmed electromyographically. The recovery of sensibility was reasonably good. The ninhydrin test showed a very slight recovery of the sweat secretion of the little finger and part of the ring finger. The two-point discrimination test gave a value of 17 to 22 mm on the volar side of the fingers and thumb.

Case 5

History: The patient, a 34 year old bricklayer, cut his left wrist to the bone in two places about 7 cm apart on the volar side and on the dorsal side in two places about 3 cm apart. On the volar side both nerves and arteries and all the tendons were severed in two places. During the primary treatment the isolated structures between the cuts were removed. For the flexor tendons this meant the removal of a piece with a length of about 3 to 5 cm, for the median nerve of 7 cm, and for the ulnar nerve of 4 cm. The arteries were ligated and the wound closed. Dorsally, only the extensor carpi ulnaris tendon was partially intact. The extensors of the fingers had been cut only once. A 3 cm long segment was removed from the tendons of the radial wrist extensors and from the thumb extensors. The extensor tendons of the fingers were sutured and the wound closed. Post-operatively, the skin did not develop necrosis. Because of the depressive state of the patient and the poor circulation in his hand, any attempt to reconstruct the function of the hand was postponed for five months.

The scar tissue situated in the volar wrist region was then excised. The defect in the deep digital flexor tendons was bridged by a single common tendon graft. The defects in the tendon of the flexor pollicis longus and the flexor carpi ulnaris were also repaired with tendon grafts. To obtain recovery of at least the protective sensibility on the radio-volar side of the hand, an attempt was made to restore the continuity of the median nerve by the nerve pedicle graft method described by Strange (1947, 1950), in which a portion of the ulnar nerve is used to repair the gap in the median. The neuromata of the median and ulnar nerves were resected and the two proximal nerve stumps anastomosed. The ulnar nerve was transected 8 cm proximal to this anastomosis, with the exception of the portion of the epineurium in which a longitudinal epineural vessel was visible; this was intended to prevent central ischaemic necrosis of the nerve if possible. Two months later, this segment of the ulnar nerve was mobilized and turned over distally to bridge the gap in the median nerve. In addition, a silastic rod was pushed subcutaneously over the thenar to the metacarpo-phalangeal joint of the thumb. A few months later the dorsal side of the wrist was explored. The defect in both radial carpal extensors was repaired by a common tendon graft, and the same was done for the defect in the abductor pollicis longus and extensor pollicis brevis tendons. The extensor pollicis longus appeared to be retracted too far. For the reconstruction of the extension of the distal phalanx of the thumb and also of a certain amount of the adductive power of the thumb, the extensor indicis proprius was transferred to the thumb and attached to the distal part of the long thumb extensor.

Examination: Eleven months after the injury, the hand had a dystrophic appearance. The intrinsic muscles were atrophic. The thumb was in extension-adduction with the distal phalanx in hyperflexion (Fig. 18). Opposition was of course impossible, the adductive power very limited. Passive mobility of the thumb was almost normal. The total flexion of the three phalanges of the fingers amounted to 100–120°. The extension of the fingers was limited to 20–40° in the proximal interphalangeal joint. The hand showed ulnar deviation in the wrist joint; radial abduction was not possible Degree and power of the wrist extension and flexion were adequate. The hand had no sensibility except in one area on the dorsal side of the thumb.

Reconstruction: For the restoration of opposition in this severe case, a choice had to be made between fixation of the thumb in opposition and a tendon transfer. Because of the excellent cooperation shown by the patient during rehabilitation exercises, preference was given to the latter. For a tendon transfer, only one suitable motor was available: the extensor proprius of the little finger. No attempt was made to determine whether the little finger could be extended when the other fingers were passively held in the completely flexed position; the consequences of this omission were later to become apparent. With respect to power, amplitude, and location, the extensor digiti quinti proprius is a reasonably good motor for the reconstruction of opposition: the tendon does not have to be lengthened and a pulley construction is not required. The extensor of the little finger was led around the ulna, drawn through the preformed pseudosheath, and then inserted on the metacarpo-phalangeal joint of the thumb according to Brand's insertion.

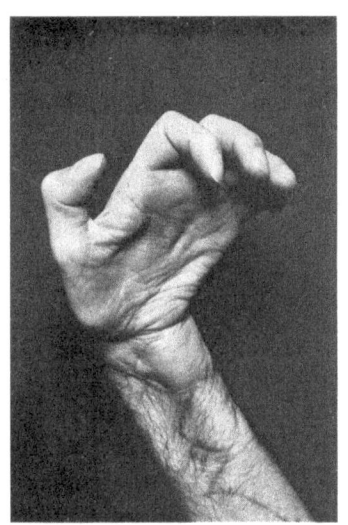

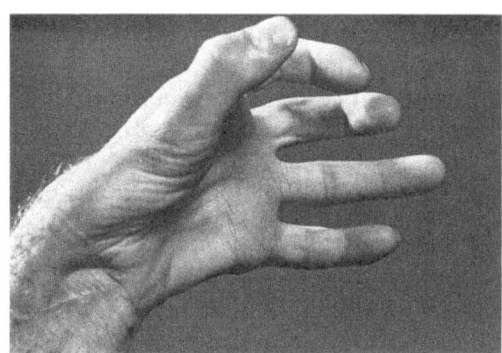

Fig. 19

Fig. 18

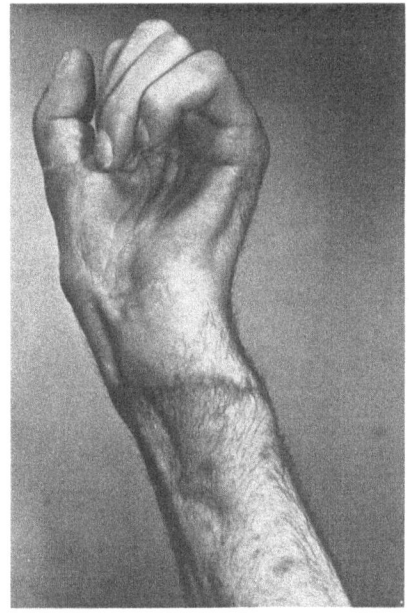

Fig. 18. Crippled hand due to an almost irreparable wrist lesion.

Fig. 19. Result of attempt to restore opposition by transfer of extensor tendon of the little finger around the ulna.

Fig. 20. Fixation of the thumb in moderate opposition by tenodesis.

Fig. 20

Results: Regarded independently, the restoration of opposition was reasonable (Fig. 19). The head of the first metacarpal could be placed opposite the shaft of the second metacarpal. The abduction distance between the thumb and the index finger was 5 cm. The thumb could reach a pronation of 30°. The proximal phalanx of the thumb was hyperextended during opposition, probably due to excessive tension on the ulnar slip of insertion. The hyperflexion of the distal phalanx was considerably reduced. Nevertheless, the patient had obtained no functional benefit at all from this opposition reconstruction. The opposition proved to act antagonistically in the grasping movement, and could only be achieved if the fingers were simultaneously extended. If the fingers were flexed, the thumb went into adduction-extension. In all probability, during the first operation performed directly after the injury the extensor digitorum communis tendon of the little finger had been sutured to the tendon of the extensor digiti quinti proprius. Although the ulnar extensor tendon of the little finger had been transferred, in actual fact a common extensor had been used as motor. The function of the fingers was appreciably improved; they could be rolled up in the palm of the hand to some extent. The most striking change was the improvement in the dystrophy of the entire hand. On the volar side of the thumb and middle finger, a certain amount of coarse sensibility was already present.

At a later date, the thumb was fixed in moderate opposition by an opponodesis and the metacarpo-phalangeal joint stabilized by an arthrodesis (Fig. 20). Seen retrospectively, this could better have been done immediately. During the intervening period, the patient was retrained for administrative work.

Case 6

History: This patient was an 18 year old window-washer who had cut himself on broken glass, causing a wound on the volar side of the right wrist The median and ulnar nerves, the radial artery, and all the flexor tendons except that of the flexor pollicis longus were severed. Primary suturing of the nerves and tendons was performed. Three weeks later, the plaster splint was replaced by a night splint to prevent an adduction contracture of the thumb (Fig. 21). A knuckle-bender splint was not required for the fingers, since the tendency to clawing was very limited.

Examination: Seven months after the accident, the radial thenar muscles were atrophic. The other intrinsic muscles showed less atrophy. The patient could only pick up small objects, such as a thin nail, with great difficulty (Fig. 22). The thumb could not be brought actively into opposition. The pinch power between thumb and index finger was one-fourth that of the left hand. The fingers showed a slight limitation of extension in the proximal interphalangeal joints, but true clawing was not present. The patient had paresthesia over the entire volar side of the hand, which is usually an indication of at least a return of protective sensibility. The electromyograms showed no distinct signs of re-innervation of the radial thenar muscles, and the other intrinsic muscles showed no greater recovery of the motor function, only the abductor digiti quinti giving a sketchy interference pattern on voluntary contraction.

Reconstruction: For the recovery of opposition, the use of an undamaged motor-tendon unit from the dorsal side of the lower arm was to be preferred. The most suitable of the dorsal muscles for this purpose were the extensor carpi ulnaris and the abductor pollicis longus, since both take part in opposition and have a favourable location for an opposition tendon transfer. Because restoration of the adductive power was also desirable in this righthanded patient and the extensor carpi ulnaris is the most suitable for an adduction tendon transfer, the abductor pollicis longus was chosen as motor for the reconstruction of opposition. The abductor longus tendon was detached at its insertion, brought around the radial side of the wrist in the volar direction, drawn under the palmaris longus tendon – as pulley – and then re-inserted slightly distal to its original site. The transferred tendon passed along the palmaris longus a few centimetres proximal to the earlier tendon suture. In preparation for the adduction tendon transfer, a silastic rod was introduced at the same time, running from the metacarpo-phalangeal joint of the thumb, under the long flexor tendons, and then via the third intermetacarpal cleft to the dorsal side of the wrist. Two months later, the rod was removed. The extensor carpi ulnaris was lengthened with a tendon graft, which was then drawn through the preformed pseudo-sheath and attached with a double insertion on the insertion of the adductor and abductor brevis.

Results: The results were surprising (Fig. 23). The abduction and flexion of the first metacarpal was equal to that of the left hand, and almost normal pronation could be achieved. There was no limitation of retroposition. The pinch power between the thumb and index finger had increased to three-fifths that of the left hand. The patient went back to work but not as a window-washer, because the sensibility of the hand was not sufficiently restored to make such work safe.

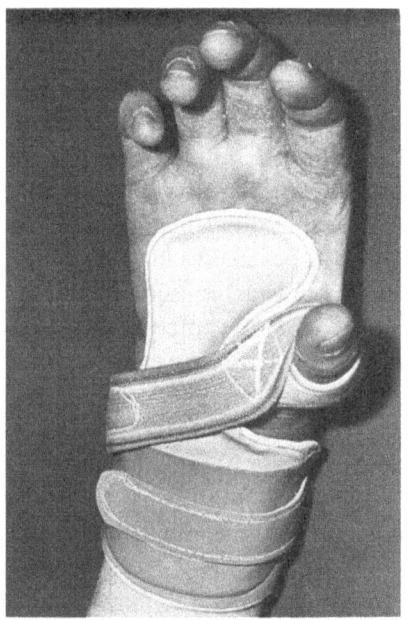

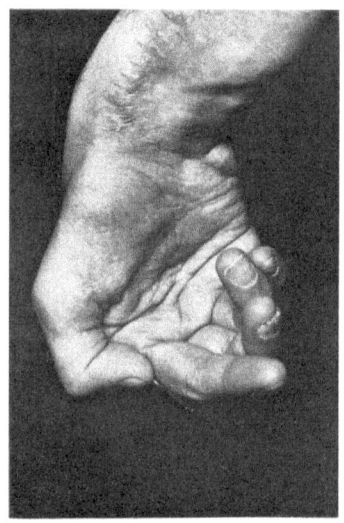

Fig. 22

Fig. 21

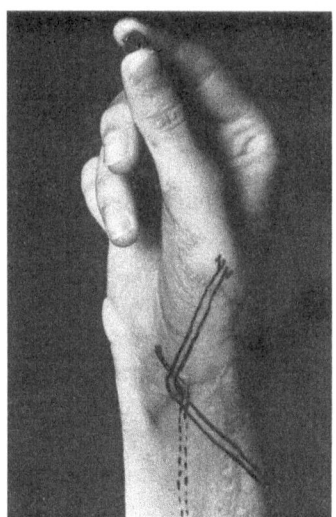

Fig. 21. Splint for thenar paralysis.

Fig. 22. Attempt at strong pinch after a median and ulnar nerve lesion.

Fig. 23. Almost normal opposition obtained by transfer of abductor pollicis longus tendon in combination with an adduction tendon transfer.

Fig. 23

DISCUSSION

Case 7

History: This patient, a 31 year old sailor, caught his right hand in an anchor winch. The skin on the dorsal side of the hand was partially destroyed. On the volar side there was a deep laceration reaching over the entire length of the thenar to the wrist. The radial thenar muscles had been torn from their origins and lay free in the wound. All the metacarpals were fractured, as were the proximal phalanges of the thumb and the little finger. Because of the severe swelling and badly contaminated wound, the initial treatment was conservative. After closure of the skin defects, open reduction of the fracture fragments was performed with fixation by means of Kirschner wires.

Examination: Four months after the accident the fractures had re-united in an acceptable position except for the base of the proximal phalanx of the thumb. There was extreme limitation of flexion of all the metacarpo-phalangeal joints. The flexion power of the fingers was about two-thirds that of the left hand. The thenar was flattened and the skin over it showed deep scarring. There was no sensibility on the radio-volar side of the thumb. Even passively, opposition was impossible. The thumb was fixed in adduction-extension. The pinch power between the thumb and index finger was appreciably lower than that of the left hand.

Reconstruction: The limitation of flexion of the metacarpo-phalangeal joints was partially abolished by a capsulolysis of these joints. The proximal phalanx of the thumb was brought into a better position by means of an arthrodesis in the metacarpo-phalangeal joint. At a subsequent operation, the adduction contracture of the thumb was corrected. Skin and fascial structures in the first metacarpal space were released. At the same time, a dorsal capsulotomy was performed on the first carpo-metacarpal joint, and the fibrotic first dorsal interosseous was excised. The insertion of the adductor was left intact. The thumb could now be brought passively into opposition and was fixed in this position by means of two Kirschner wires (Fig. 24). The skin defect was repaired with a pedicle flap from the thorax. Since the scarring of the thenar ran through the line of pull of an opposition tendon transfer, a silastic rod was introduced under

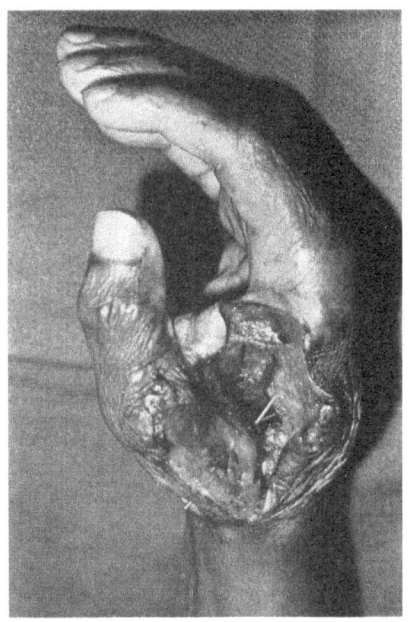

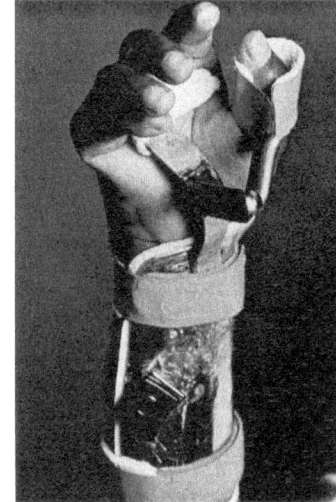

Fig. 25

Fig. 24

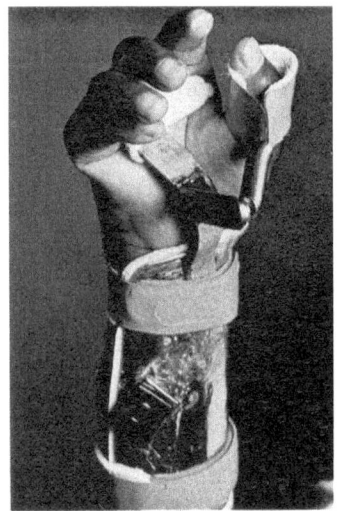

Fig. 26

Fig. 24. Correction of a severe adduction contracture.

Fig. 25. Powerful dynamic splint to maintain the restored abduction position.

Fig. 26. Restoration of opposition by transfer of extensor carpi ulnaris tendon through a preformed pseudosheath.

the scarred area. When the pedicle flap had been completely transferred to the first intermetacarpal space, the Kirschner wires were removed and a powerful dynamic splint was applied to maintain the abduction position reached for the thumb (Fig. 25).

Two months later, the mobility of the first carpo-metacarpal joint was sufficiently restored to permit reconstruction of the opposition by means of a tendon transfer. Because of the reduced flexion power of the fingers, transfer of one of the superficial flexor tendons was contra-indicated. Transfer of the abductor longus tendon could not be considered because of the scarring around the insertion of the palmaris longus. Tansfer of the abductor digiti quinti to the scarred thenar region involved too much risk. The extensor carpi ulnaris was therefore chosen as motor, which made it possible to avoid a pulley mechanism in the scarred wrist region. The silastic rod was removed, and the wrist extensor was lengthened with a tendon transplant, which was led in the volar direction around the ulna, through the preformed tunnel, and then attached to the insertion of the abductor pollicis brevis.

Results: The opposition of the thumb was satisfactory (Fig. 26). The maximal abduction distance between the distal flexion crease of the thumb and the base of the index finger was 6 cm. The flexion of the first metacarpal was adequate, but its head could not be placed opposite the third metacarpal. The total flexion-extension movement of the first metacarpal amounted to 35° (*versus* 50° in the left hand). There was no limitation of adduction. Although the total rotation movement of the thumb was limited, the pronation position in opposition was good, perhaps even with some overcompensation by the arthrodesis of the metacarpo-phalangeal joint. The movement of the distal phalanx of the thumb was normal. Thirteen months after the accident the patient was working in the harbour, but he was no longer suitable for his original occupation.

Case 8

History: This patient was a child with a floating thumb on the right hand. The hypoplastic thumb, which had two phalanges and a nail, was attached by a narrow pedicle. The first metacarpal was lacking. At the age of five months, the vestigial thumb was removed and pollicization of the index finger was performed (Fig. 27). Intrinsic thumb muscles and the tendons of the extrinsic thumb muscles were found to be absent as well as the trapezium and scaphoid bones. After an osteotomy just proximal to the head of the second metacarpal, the index finger with the head of the second metacarpal was transposed to the thumb position. The head of the second metacarpal was fixed on the radio-volar side of the base of the same metacarpal. The flexor and extensor tendons of the reconstructed thumb were not shortened. The first dorsal and volar interossei were inserted more distally in the extensor aponeurosis of the new thumb in order to retain the abductive and adductive action of these muscles.

Examination: Fig. 28 shows the reconstructed thumb, nine months after the pollicization. The thumb was used for grasping as a contrafinger, but the abduction was not entirely adequate and the pronation was also limited. The flexion and extension could be considered normal. Due to the limited abduction and pronation of the thumb, the child picked up small objects between the volar side of the distal thumb phalanx and the radial side of the distal phalanx of the middle finger. Thus, precision handling was hampered. In a child of this age it was difficult to measure the adductive power of the reconstructed thumb, but it was estimated to be between one-fourth and one-third that of the normal left thumb.

Reconstruction: This was a case of incomplete opposition of the thumb, which is basically a minor anomaly preferably corrected by a simple reconstruction. In this case transfer of the abductor digiti quinti or the tendon of a wrist extensor or superficial finger flexor would have given a gain of opposition at the almost equal cost of a secondary functional loss. Furthermore, a powerful motor was not required to improve opposition. The palmaris longus tendon could be palpated, and transfer of this tendon seemed to be the most suitable procedure for this case. The palmaris longus was detached from its insertion, leaving a strip of the palmar fascia about 2 cm long on the tendon. This strip was inserted on the base of the proximal phalanx ('metacarpal') of the reconstructed thumb. A pulley mechanism was not required, since the object was only to correct the abduction and possibly also the pronation, since the thumb could be flexed normally.

Results: Six weeks after the transfer the abduction of the thumb was normal and the pronation showed some improvement. Precision handling could be adequately performed (Fig. 29).

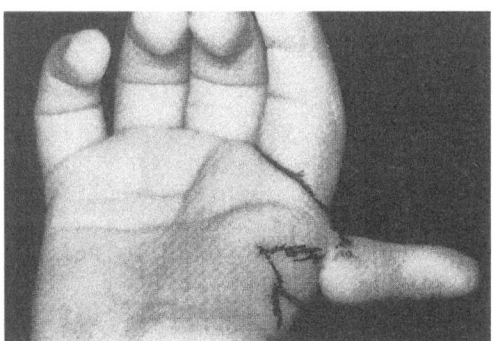

Fig. 27

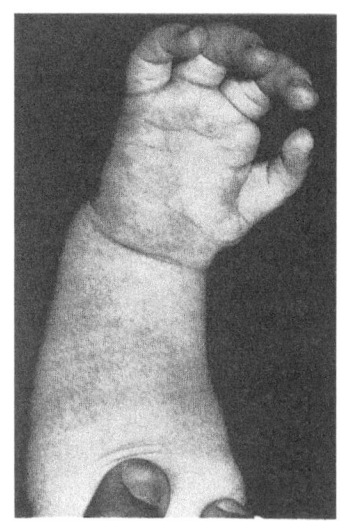

Fig. 28

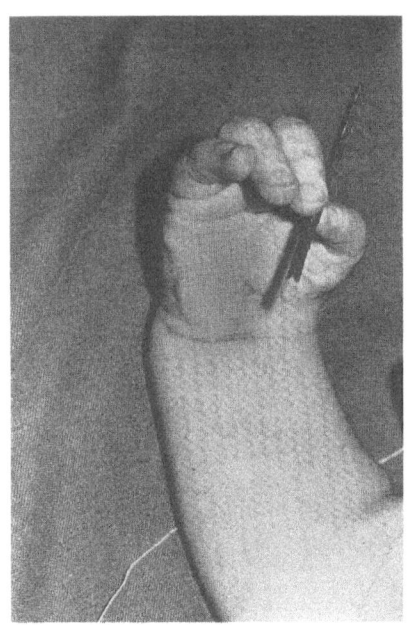

Fig. 29

Fig. 27. Floating thumb.

Fig. 28. Pollicization of the index finger.

Fig. 29. Opposition improved by transfer of palmaris longus tendon.

CONCLUSIONS

A dynamic reconstruction of the lost opposition of the thumb can be achieved in several ways, the methods differing in the choice of the motor, the use of a pulley, and the manner of insertion.

The motor: Transfer of the abductor digiti quinti is a very effective method in cases of an isolated median paralysis, but is not without hazard. Almost all the extrinsic muscles of the lower arm can also be used as motor, the most suitable being the flexor superficialis of the ring finger, the extensor carpi ulnaris, and the abductor pollicis longus – the last, however, only in cases of a combined median and ulnar paralysis. The flexor digitorum profundus, the flexor carpi ulnaris, and the brachioradialis are less suitable, and the extensor digitorum communis and the extensor pollicis longus are not suitable at all. Which muscle can best be chosen in a given case is dependent on the nature and extent of the paralysis or lesion, the functional dispensability of the muscle in the particular case, and the presence of scar tissue. The power and amplitude of the motor are of secondary importance for the reconstruction of opposition.

The pulley: In cases with paralysis of all the intrinsic muscles, the transferred tendon should pull from the vicinity of the pisiform bone. If the main problem is limited to restricted abduction of the thumb (incomplete opposition), the pull should come from a more radially situated point. In most cases a fulcrum or pulley is required to give the tendon the correct direction of pull. There are at least ten possibilities for the establishment of a pulley, the most important factor being the location. The pulley mechanism itself is less essential. A good pulley possibility is offered by the tendon of the flexor carpi ulnaris or the ulnar edge of the ulna. If deep scarring is present in the wrist region, it is sometimes possible to choose a pulley situated such that the transferred tendon need not be led through the scar tissue. If this is not possible, a silastic rod can be introduced into the scarred region; upon removal of the rod a few months later, the tendon can be transferred through the preformed pseudosheath. With this method the development of adhesions around the transferred tendon is appreciably reduced.

The insertion: The insertion of the transferred tendon is the only step in the reconstruction of opposition for which a standard procedure can be applied. In cases of paralysis of the radial thenar muscles an attachment to the abductor pollicis brevis insertion is used. When all the intrinsic thumb muscles are paralysed, the metacarpo-phalangeal joint of the thumb must be stabilized as well; this can be done most effectively by the insertion according to Brand. If, in cases of median and ulnar paralysis, the abductor longus is transferred and inserted at the base of the first metacarpal, the metacarpo-phalangeal joint should be stabilized by capsuloplasty, arthrodesis, or an adduction tendon transfer.

SUMMARY

The grasp function of the hand is dependent on the ability to place the thumb opposite the fingers. The opposition of the thumb is described as a complex of fundamental movements in the three distal thumb joints in which all the intrinsic and extrinsic muscles of the thumb are involved.

The functional disturbances accompanying paralysis of the thenar muscles are discussed. A distinction is made between disturbance of the power grip and disturbance of precision handling, the loss of opposition of the thumb being important in both.

A dynamic restoration of the lost opposition can be achieved by the transfer of an intrinsic muscle or transfer of the tendon of an extrinsic muscle. For the tendon approach, many transfer possibilities are available. Some of these afford adequate compensation for a paralysis of the radial thenar muscles, others are less effective in this respect. Because of the great disparity in the nature and extent of the paralysis or of the damage resulting from the injury, it is often impossible to apply a standard procedure. For each opposition reconstruction a choice must be made from a wide range of transfer possibilities. The present paper offers a survey of the data relevant to this choice. A review of the various approaches to the reconstruction of opposition is given, as well as an analysis of the elements involved: the motor, the fulcrum, and the insertion. The factors to be considered in the choice of a suitable transfer method are discussed in detail.

The most important aspects of the recovery of opposition are elucidated on the basis of a number of selected cases.

Acknowledgements

I wish to express my gratitude to Dr. J. C. Raadsveld, who trained
me in plastic surgery and gave me the opportunity to prepare this
thesis.

My thanks for valuable assistance are extended to Mr. J. W.
Wesseling, Head of the Department of Medical Photography of the
Rotterdam Faculty of Medicine, and his assistants, in particular
Mr. S. M. László and Mr. T. van de Biessen; Miss A. P. Wegter
and S. M. van Loon of the Medical Library; and to Mrs. I. Seeger,
who translated the text.

LITERATURE

Adam, R.: *La restauration du mouvement d'opposition du pouce*, Thesis, Paris, 1941.

Baeyer, H. von: Translokation von Sehnen, *Z. orthop. Chir.* 56: 552, 1932.

Bassett, C. A. L., and Carroll, R. E.: Formation of tendon sheath by silicone-rod implants, *J. Bone Jt Surg.* 45-A: 884, 1963.

Baumann, J. A.: Valeur, variations et equivalences des muscles extenseurs, interosseux, adducteur set abducteurs de la main et du pied, chez l'homme, *Acta anat.* 4: 10, 1947.

Berg, J. H. van den: *Metabletica van de materie*, G. F. Callenbach N.V., Nijkerk, p. 101 and 423, 1969.

Björkesten, G. af: Position of fingers and function deficiency in ulnar paralysis, *Acta chir. scand.* 93: 99, 1946.

Bohr, H. H.: Tendon transposition in paralysis of the opposition of the thumb, *Acta chir. scand.* 105: 45, 1953.

Bowden, R. E. M., and Napier, J. R.: The assessment of hand function after peripheral nerve injuries, *J. Bone Jt Surg.* 43-B: 481, 1961.

Boyes, J. H.: Selection of a donor muscle for tendon transfer, *J. Hosp. Jt Dis.* 23: 1, 1962.

Boyes, J. H.: *Bunnell's Surgery of the hand*, J. B. Lippincott Co., Philadelpia, 1964.

Brand, P. W.: Tendon grafting, illustrated by a new operation for intrinsic paralysis of the fingers, *J. Bone Jt Surg.* 43-B: 444, 1961.

Brand, P. W.: The hand in leprosy, in *Clinical surgery, The hand*, ed. R. G. Pulvertaft, Butterworths, London, p. 279, 1966.

Brooks, D.M.: Inter-metacarpal bone graft for thenar paralysis, *J. Bone Jt Surg.* 31-B: 511, 1949.

Brooks, D. M.: Treatment of the paralytic hand, in *Clinical surgery, The hand*, ed. R. G. Pulvertaft, Butterworths, London, p. 269, 1966.

Bunnell, S.: Reconstructive surgery of the hand, *Surg. Gynec. Obstet.* 39: 259, 1924.

Bunnell, S.: Opposition of the thumb, *J. Bone Jt Surg.* 20: 269, 1938.

Bunnell, S.: Surgery of the intrinsic muscles of the hand other than those producing opposition of the thumb, *J. Bone Jt Surg.* 24: 1, 1942.

Bunnell, S.: *Surgery of the hand*, J. B. Lippincott Co., Philadelphia, 3rd ed., 1956.

Camitz, H.: Über die Behandlung der Oppositionslähmung, *Acta chir. scand.* 65: 77, 1929.

Carayon, A., Bourrel, P., Languillon, J., and Boissan, R. H.: Opération poulie et opération de Steindler dans la restauration de l'opposition du pouce chez le lépreux, *Rev. Chir. orthop.* 48: 259, 1962.

Cliffton, E. E.: Unusual innervation of the intrinsic muscles of the hand by median and ulnar nerves, *Surgery* 23: 12, 1948.

Coeur, P. le: Procédé de restauration de l'opposition du pouce par transplantation sur chevalet, *Rev. Chir. orthop.* 39: 655, 1953.

Colville, J., Callison, J. R., and White, W. L.: Role of mesotenon in tendon blood supply, *Plast. reconstr. Surg.* 43: 53, 1969.

Day, M. H., and Napier, J. R.: The two heads of flexor pollicis brevis, *J. Anat. (Lond.)* 95: 123, 1961.

Deyerle, W. M., and Tucker, F.: Tendon transplants in the wrist following nerve injury, *Sth. med. J.* 53: 1562, 1960.

Duchenne, G. B. A.: *Physiology of motion*; translated by E. B. Kaplan, W. B. Saunders Co., Philadelphia/London, 1959.

Edgerton, M. T., Snyder, G. B., and Webb, W. L.: Surgical treatment of congenital thumb deformities, *J. Bone Jt Surg.* 47-A: 1453, 1965.

Edgerton, M. T., and Brand, P. W.: Restoration of abduction and adduction to the unstable thumb in median and ulnar paralysis, *Plast. reconstr. Surg.* 36: 150, 1965.

Fenton, R. L., and Lapidus, P. W.: An anatomical study of the abductor pollicis longus and extensor pollicis longus and brevis, *Bull. Hosp. Jt Dis.* 14: 138, 1953.

Fick, R.: *Handbuch der Anatomie und Mechanik der Gelenke III*, G. Fischer, Jena, 1911.

Flynn, J. E., and Flynn, W. F.: Median and ulnar nerve injuries; a long range study with evaluation of the ninhydrin test, sensory and motor returns, *Ann. Surg.* 156: 1002, 1962.

Foerster, O.: Beitrag zum Werte fixierender orthopädischer Operationen bei Nervenkrankheiten, *Acta chir. scand.* 67: 351, 1930.

Forrest, W. J., and Basmajian, J. V.: Functions of human thenar and hypothenar muscles, *J. Bone Jt Surg.* 47-A: 1585, 1965.

Göbell, R., and Freudenberg, K.: Guter Operationserfolg durch Transplantation des Flexor dig. subl. V bei Opponensaplasie des Daumens, *Arch. orthop. Unfall-Chir.* 35: 675, 1935.

Goldner, J. L., and Irwin, C. E.: An analysis of paralytic thumb deformities, *J. Bone Jt Surg.* 32-A: 627, 1950.

Goldner, J. L.: Reconstructive surgery of the hand in cerebral palsy and spastic paralysis resulting from injury to the spinal cord, *J. Bone Jt Surg.* 37-A: 1141, 1955.

Goldner, J. L., and Clippinger, F. W.: Excision of the greater multangular bone as an adjunct to mobilization of the thumb, *J. Bone Jt Surg.* 41-A: 609, 1959.

Grünkorn, J.: Die Daumenopposition, ihre muskelphysiologische Erklärung und die Behandlung des Oppositionsausfalls, *Z. orthop. Chir.* 57: 517, 1932.

Hage, J.: *Het tot duim maken van de wijsvinger volgens Littler*, Thesis, Groningen, 1966.

Haines, R. W.: The mechanism of rotation at the first carpo-metacarpal joint, *J. Anat. (Lond.)* 78: 44, 1944.

Hakstian, R. W.: Funicular orientation by direct stimulation; an aid to peripheral nerve repair, *J. Bone Jt Surg.* 50-A: 1178, 1968.

Harris, H. A., and Joseph, H.: Variation in extension of the metacarpo-phalangeal and interphalangeal joints of the thumb, *J. Bone Jt Surg.* 31-B: 547, 1949.

Harrison, S. H.: Restoration of muscle balance in pollicization, *Plast. reconstr. Surg.* 34: 236, 1964.

Hass, J.: Zur Sehnenoperation bei Medianuslähmung, *Zbl. Chir.* 28: 532, 1919.

Henderson, E. D.: Transfer of wrist extensors and brachioradialis to restore opposition of the thumb, *J. Bone Jt Surg.* 44-A: 513, 1962.

Hettinger, T.: *Physiology of strength*, ed. M. H. Thurlwell, C. C. Thomas, Springfield, Illinois, p. 12, 1961.

Holevich, J.: A new method of restoring sensibility to the thumb, *J. Bone Jt Surg.* 45-B: 496, 1963.

Howell, B. W.: A new operation for opponens paralysis of the thumb, *Lancet,* 1: 131, 1926.

Huber, E.: Hilfsoperation bei Medianuslähmung, *Dtsch. Z. Chir.* 162: 271, 1921.

Hueston, J. T.: A combined sensory and motor transfer for median lesions, *Brit. J. plast. Surg.* 20: 385, 1967.

Huffstadt, A. J. C., and Bom, A. W.: Verdere ervaringen met de pollicisatie-operatie, *Ned. T. Geneesk.* 104: 1760, 1960.

Iselin, M.: *Chirurgie de la main,* Masson et Cie, Paris, 2nd ed., p. 314, 1955.

Jacobs, B., and Thompson, T. C.: Opposition of the thumb and its restoration, *J. Bone Jt Surg.* 42-A: 1015, 1960.

Jahn, A.: Aktiver Ersatz bei Oppositionslähmung des Daumens, *Z. orthop. Chir.* 51: 100, 1929.

Jones, F. W.: *Principles of anatomy as seen in the hand,* Baillière, Tindall and Cox, London, 2nd ed., 1944.

Jones, W. B., and Goldner, J. L.: Anomalous innervation of the forearm and hand, *J. Bone Jt Surg.* 48-A: 604, 1966.

Joseph, J.: Further studies of the metacarpo-phalangeal and interphalangeal joints of the thumb, *J. Anat. (Lond.)* 85: 221, 1951.

Joseph, J.: The sesamoid bones of the hand and the time of fusion of the epiphyses of the thumb, *J. Anat. (Lond.)* 85: 230, 1951.

Kaneff, A.: Über die wechselseitigen Beziehungen der progressiven Merkmale des M. extensor pollicis brevis beim Menschen, *Anat. Anz.* 122: 31, 1968.

Kaplan, E. B.: *Functional and surgical anatomy of the hand,* J. B. Lippincott Co., Philadelphia, 2nd ed., 1965.

Kirklin, J. W., and Thomas, C. G.: Opponens transplant; an analysis of the methods employed and results obtained in seventy-five cases, *Surg. Gynec. Obstet.* 86: 213, 1948.

Kochs: Opponens-Plastik, *Chirurg* 4: 67, 1932.

Krukenberg, H.: Ueber Ersatz des M. opponens pollicis, *Z. orthop. Chir.* 42: 178, 1921.

Landsmeer, J. M. F.: Anatomical and functional investigations of the articulation of the human fingers, *Acta anat., suppl.* 24, 1955.

Landsmeer, J. M. F.: Power grip and precision handling, *Ann. rheum. Dis.* 21: 164, 1962.

Landsmeer, J. M. F.: Personal communication, 1969.

Lange, F.: Die Sehnenverpflanzung, *Ergebn. Chir. Orthop.* 2: 1, 1911.

Lange, M.: Die Behandlung der irreparablen peripheren Nervenverletzungen, *Wiederherstellungschir. u. Traum* 1: 240, 1953.

Lanz, T. von, Wachsmuth, W.: *Praktische Anatomie,* Arm, Springer, Berlin, 1959.

Littler, J. W.: Tendon transfers and arthrodeses in combined median and ulnar nerve paralysis, *J. Bone Jt Surg.* 31-A: 225, 1949.

Littler, J. W.: Neurovascular skin island transfer in reconstructive hand surgery, *Transact. Int. Soc. Plast. Surg.,* 2nd Congr. London 1959, Ed. A. B. Wallace, Livingstone, Edinburgh, p. 175, 1960.

Littler, J. W.: The physiology and dynamic function of the hand, *Surg. Clin. N. Amer.* 40: 259, 1960.

Littler, J. W., and Cooley, S. G. E.: Opposition of the thumb and its restoration by abductor digiti quinti transfer, *J. Bone Jt Surg.* 45-A: 1389, 1963.

Littler, J. W., and Li, C. S.: Primary restoration of thumb opposition with median nerve decompression, *Plast. reconstr. Surg.* 39: 74, 1967.

Lipscomb, P. R., Elkins, E. C., and Henderson, E. D.: Tendon transfers to restore function of hands in tetraplegia, especially after fracture-dislocation of the sixth cervical vertebra on the seventh, *J. Bone Jt Surg.* 40-A: 1071, 1958.

Luckey, C. A., and McPherson, S. R.: Tendinous reconstruction of the hand following irreparable injury to the peripheral nerves and brachial plexus, *J. Bone Jt Surg.* 29: 560, 1947.

MacConaill, M. A.: Studies in the mechanics of synovial joints; fundamental principles and diadochal movements, *Irish J. med. Sci.* 246: 190, 1946.

MacConaill, M. A.: Studies in the mechanics of synovial joints; displacements of articular surfaces and the significance of saddle joints, *Irish J. med. Sci.* 247: 223, 1946.

Makin, M.: Translocation of the flexor pollicis longus tendon to restore opposition, *J. Bone Jt Surg.* 49-B: 458, 1967.

Mangini, U.: Flexor pollicis longus muscle; its morphology and clinical significance, *J. Bone Jt Surg.* 42-A: 467, 1960.

Mangini, U.: Dynamic and static recovery of opposition of the thumb; operative techniques and their indications, *Panmin. Med.* 10: 152, 1968.

Mannerfelt, L.: Studies on the hand in ulnar nerve paralysis; a clinical-experimental investigation in normal and anomalous innervation, *Acta orthop. scand.*, *suppl.* 87, 1966.

Matev, I.: Réhabilitation fonctionelle du pouce dans une paralysie cubitale basse irréductible, *Ann. Chir. plast.* 5: 23, 1960.

Mayer, L.: The physiological method of tendon transplantation; operative technique, *Surg. Gynec. Obstet.* 22: 298, 1916.

Mayer, L., and Ransohoff, N.: Reconstruction of the digital tendon sheath; a contribution to the physiological method of repair of damaged finger tendons, *J. Bone Jt Surg.* 18: 607, 1936.

McFarlane, R. M.: Observations on the functional anatomy of the intrinsic muscles of the thumb, *J. Bone Jt Surg.* 44-A: 1073, 1962.

Meulen, J. C. H. van der: To be published.

Milgram, J. E.: Transplantation of tendons through preformed gliding channels, *Bull. Hosp. Jt Dis.* 21: 250, 1960.

Moberg, E.: Methods for examining sensibility of the hand, in *Hand surgery*, ed. J. E. Flynn, Williams and Wilkins Co., Baltimore, p. 435, 1966.

Moberg, E.: Nerve repair in hand surgery, an analysis, *Surg. Clin. N. Amer.* 48: 985, 1968.

Moberg, E.: In: Bericht über das 8. Symposium der deutschsprachigen Arbeitsgemeinschaft für Handchirurgie, Wien 1968, *Handchir.* 2: 74, 1969.

Murphey, F., Kirklin, J. W., and Finlayson, A. I.: Anomalous innervation of the instrinsic muscles of the hand, *Surg. Gynec. Obstet.* 83: 15, 1946.

Napier, J. R.: The attachments and function of the abductor pollicis brevis, *J. Anat. (Lond.)* 86: 335, 1952.

Napier, J. R.: The form and function of the carpo-metacarpal joint of the thumb, *J. Anat. (Lond.)* 89: 362, 1955.

Ney, K. W.: A tendon transplant for intrinsic hand muscle paralysis, *Surg. Gynec. Obstet.* 33: 342, 1921.

Nicholson, O. R., and Seddon, H. J.: Nerve repair in civil practice, Results of treatment of median and ulnar nerve lesions, *Brit. med. J.* 2: 5053, 1957.

Nicoladoni: Nachtrag zur Pes calcaneus und zur Transplantation der Peronealsehnen, *Arch. klin. Chir.* 27: 660, 1882.

Nicolaysen, J.: In *Nordisk Kirurgisk Forenung Förhandlingar*, 13th Meeting, Helsingfors, p. 118, 1921.

Nicolaysen, J.: Transplantation des M. abductor dig. V bei fehlender Oppositionsfähigkeit des Daumens, *Dtsch. Z. Chir.* 168: 133, 1922.

Nielsen, P. H.: Tendon transplantation for the repair of opponens paralysis of the thumb, *Acta orthop. scand.* 16: 148, 1946.

Önne, L.: Recovery of sensibility and sudomotor activity in the hand after nerve suture, *Acta chir. scand., suppl.* 300, 1962.

Palazzi, A. S.: On the treatment of the loss of opposition, *Acta orthop. scand.* 32: 396, 1962.

Phalen, G. S., and Miller, R. C.: The transfer of wrist extensor muscles to restore or reinforce flexion power of the fingers and opposition of the thumb, *J. Bone Jt Surg.* 29: 993, 1947.

Price, E. W.: A two-tendon transplant for low median-ulnar palsy of the thumb in leprosy, *Proc. roy. Soc. Med.* 61: 220, 1968.

Rabischong, P.: Anatomie fonctionelle de l'opposition du pouce, Groupe d'étude de la chirurgie de la main, Nov. 28, 1964.

Rowntree, T.: Anomalous innervation of the hand muscles, *J. Bone Jt Surg.* 31-B: 505, 1949.

Royle, N. D.: An operation for paralysis of the intrinsic muscles of the thumb, *J. Amer. med. Ass.* 111: 612, 1938.

Scherb, R.: Über den Ersatz poliomyelitisch gelähmter Daumenmuskeln durch Sehnentransplantation und über das Fehlen antagonistischer Bindungen an der oberen Extremität, *Schweiz. med. Wschr.* 75: 744, 1945.

Schink, W.: Zur chirurgischen Behandlung der kombinierten Medianus- und Ulnarislähmung, *Langenbecks Arch. klin. Chir.* 299: 748, 1962.

Schmidt, R., Schultka, R., Hammer, R., and Dorn, A.: Untersuchungen zur Häufigkeit accessorischer Sehnen des M. abductor pollicis longus unter Berücksichtigung ihrer Bedeutung für die Praxis, *Gegenbaurs morph. Jb.* 112: 139, 1968.

Silfverskiöld, N.: Sehnentransplantationsmethode bei Lähmung der Oppositionsfähigkeit des Daumens, *Acta chir. scand.* 64: 296, 1928.

Smith, J. W., and Conway, H.: La dynamique du glissement des tendons normaux et greffés, *Rev. Chir. orthop.* 52: 185, 1966.

Spitzy, H.: Hand und Fingerplastiken (Referat zum 14. Orthop. Kongr., Wien, 1918), *Verhandl. deutsch. orthop. Ges.* 14: 120, 1919.

Starr, C. L.: Army experience with tendon transference, *J. Bone Jt Surg.* 4: 3, 1922.

Stein, A. H. Jr.: Variations of the tendons of insertion of the abductor pollicis longus and the extensor pollicis brevis, *Anat. Rec.* 110: 49, 1951.

Steindler, A.: Orthopedic operations on the hand, *J. Amer. med. Ass.* 71: 1288, 1918.

Steindler, A.: Flexor plasty of the thumb in thenar palsy, *Surg. Gynec. Obstet.* 50: 1005, 1930.

90   LITERATURE

Strange, F. G. S. C.: An operation for nerve pedicle grafting; preliminary communi-
cation, *Brit. J. Surg.* 34: 423, 1947.
Strange, F. G. S. C.: Case report on pedicled nerve-graft, *Brit. J. Surg.* 37: 331, 1950.
Sunderland, S.: *Nerves and nerve injuries*, E. and S. Livingstone Ltd., Edinburgh and
London, p. 683, 1968.

Taylor, R. T.: Reconstruction of the hand, *Surg. Gynec. Obstet.* 32: 237, 1921.
Thompson, C. F.: Fusion of the metacarpals of the thumb and index finger to maintain
functional position of the thumb, *J. Bone Jt Surg.* 24: 907, 1942.
Thompson, T. C.: A modified operation for opponens paralysis, *J. Bone Jt Surg.* 24:
632, 1942.
Tubiana, R., and Lord, G.: Contractures et paralysies des muscles intrinsèques de la
main, *Ann. Chir.* 31: 285, 1955.
Tubiana, R., and Valentin, P.: Opposition of the thumb, *Surg. Clin. N. Amer.* 48:
967, 1968.

Valentin, P.: Anatomie fonctionelle des muscles de la main, *S.I.C.O.T.*, 10th Congr.
Paris 1966, ed. M. J. Delchef, Acta Medica Belgica, Brussels, p. 883, 1967.

Wells, K. F.: *Kinesiology*, W. B. Saunders Co., Philadelphia and London, 2nd ed.,
p. 22, 1955.
White, W. L.: Restoration of function and balance of the wrist and hand by tendon
transfers, *Surg. Clin. N. Amer.* 40: 427, 1960.
White, W. L.: In: Discussion on paper of E. D. Henderson, *J. Bone Jt Surg.* 44-A:
513, 1962.
Williams, S. B.: New dynamic concepts in the grafting of flexor tendons, *Plast. reconstr.
Surg.* 36: 377, 1965.
Williams, H. W. G.: The leprosy thumb, *Brit. J. plast, Surg.* 19: 136, 1966.

Zachary, R. B.: Results of nerve suture, in *Peripheral nerve injuries*, ed. H. J. Seddon,
Med. Res. Counc. Spec. Rep. Ser. no. 282, H. M. Stationery Office, London,
p. 354, 1954.
Zancolli, E.: Tendon transfers after ischemic contracture of the forearm, *Amer. J.
Surg.* 109: 356, 1965.
Zancolli, E.: *Structural and dynamic bases of hand surgery*, J. B. Lippincott Co.,
Philadelphia, p. 26, 1968.
Zrubecky, G.: Die operative Wiederherstellung des Spitzgriffes bei einer irreversiblen
Ulnarislähmung, *Arch. orthop. Unfall-Chir.* 51: 582, 1960.